TECHNICAL REPORT

National Evaluation of Safe Start Promising Approaches

Assessing Program Outcomes

Lisa H. Jaycox • Laura J. Hickman • Dana Schultz • Dionne Barnes-Proby
Claude Messan Setodji • Aaron Kofner • Racine Harris • Joie D. Acosta • Taria Francois

Sponsored by the U.S. Department of Justice's Office of Juvenile Justice and Delinquency Prevention

RAND

HEALTH and
INFRASTRUCTURE, SAFETY, AND ENVIRONMENT

This research was sponsored by the U.S. Department of Justice's Office of Juvenile Justice and Delinquency Prevention and was conducted under the auspices of the Safety and Justice Program within RAND Infrastructure, Safety, and Environment and under RAND Health's Health Promotion and Disease Prevention Program.

Library of Congress Control Number: 2011935596

ISBN: 978-0-8330-5822-5

Published 2011 by the RAND Corporation
1776 Main Street, P.O. Box 2138, Santa Monica, CA 90407-2138
1200 South Hayes Street, Arlington, VA 22202-5050
4570 Fifth Avenue, Suite 600, Pittsburgh, PA 15213-2665
RAND URL: http://www.rand.org/
To order RAND documents or to obtain additional information, contact
Distribution Services: Telephone: (310) 451-7002;
Fax: (310) 451-6915; Email: order@rand.org

Preface

Safe Start Promising Approaches (SSPA) is the second phase of a planned four-phase initiative focusing on preventing and reducing the impact of children's exposure to violence (CEV). This project was supported by Grant Nos. 2005-JW-BX-0001 and 2009-IJ-CX-0072, awarded by the Office of Juvenile Justice and Delinquency Prevention (OJJDP), Office of Justice Programs, U.S. Department of Justice. Points of view or opinions in this document are those of the authors and do not necessarily represent the official position or policies of the U.S. Department of Justice. The RAND Corporation conducted the national evaluation of the SSPA phase of the initiative in collaboration with the national evaluation team: OJJDP, the Safe Start Center, the Association for the Study and Development of Communities (ASDC), and the 15 program sites. The evaluation design involved three components: an outcomes evaluation; a process evaluation, including a cost analysis; and an evaluation of training.

This document provides the results of the outcomes evaluation, supplemented from the previous version of this report after funding was made available to analyze additional data collected at four of the original 15 sites. In the main body of this report we provide information on the designs of the studies, instruments used, data collection and cleaning, analytic methods, and an overview of the results across the 15 sites. In the appendixes, we provide a detailed description of the outcome evaluation conducted at each SSPA program, including a description of the enrollees, enrollment and retention, the amount and type of services received, and child and family-level outcomes over time.

These results will be of interest to researchers, clinicians, practitioners, policymakers, community leaders, and others interested in evaluating and implementing programs for children exposed to violence.

This research was conducted under the auspices of the Safety and Justice Program within RAND Infrastructure, Safety, and Environment (ISE) and under RAND Health's Health Promotion and Disease Prevention Program.

The mission of RAND Infrastructure, Safety, and Environment is to improve the development, operation, use, and protection of society's essential physical assets and natural resources and to enhance the related social assets of safety and security of individuals in transit and in their workplaces and communities. Safety and Justice Program research addresses occupational safety, transportation safety, food safety, and public safety—including violence, policing, corrections, substance abuse, and public integrity. Information about the Safety and Justice Program is available online (http://www.rand.org/ise/safety).

RAND Health, a division within RAND, is one of the largest private health research groups in the world. The projects within RAND Health address a wide range of health care policy issues; the agenda emphasizes policy research that can improve the health of people around the world. This project was conducted within the RAND Health Promotion and Disease Prevention Program (HPDP). RAND HPDP addresses issues related to measuring healthy and unhealthy behaviors, examining the distribution of health behaviors across population subgroups, identifying what causes or influences such behaviors, and designing and evaluating interventions to improve health behaviors. A profile of the Health division, abstracts of its publications, and ordering information can be found at www.rand.org/health.

Contents

Figures

Tables

Summary

Background

Nationally, approximately 61 percent of children have been exposed to violence during the past year, and there is reason to believe that the problem has grown worse in recent decades (Finkelhor et al., 2009). Children's exposure to violence (CEV) can have serious consequences, including a variety of psychiatric disorders and behavioral problems, such as posttraumatic stress disorder (PTSD), depression, and anxiety. School performance has also been shown to suffer as a result. Moreover, research suggests that the effects of exposure to violence may persist well into adulthood (Margolin and Gordis, 2000). Though some research has shown that early childhood interventions can substantially improve children's chances of future social and psychological well-being, many such programs have not been evaluated to date, and still others have not been examined in real-world community settings. This report presents data that were gathered in experimental and quasi-experimental studies conducted to attempt to fill these gaps in understanding about the effectiveness of programs intended to improve outcomes for children exposed to violence.

Safe Start Promising Approaches (SSPA) is one phase of a community-based initiative focused on developing and fielding interventions to prevent and reduce the impact of CEV. Sponsored by the U.S. Department of Justice's Office of Juvenile Justice and Delinquency Prevention (OJJDP), the Safe Start Initiative consists of four phases:

- Phase One: This phase focuses on expanding the system of care for children exposed to violence by conducting demonstration projects. Now complete, this phase involved demonstrations of various innovative promising practices in the system of care for children who have been exposed to violence.
- Phase Two: Building on Phase One, this phase was intended to implement and evaluate promising and evidence-based programs in community settings to identify how well programs worked in reducing and preventing the harmful effects of CEV on children.
- Phase Three: Still in the planning stages, the aim of this phase is to build a knowledge base of effective interventions in the field of CEV.
- Phase Four: The goal of this phase is to "seed" on a national scale the effective strategies identified in the earlier phases.

Each phase also includes an evaluation component that is intended to assess the implementation of the various interventions and their impact on children's outcomes.

This report focuses on Phase Two of the Safe Start Initiative. For this phase, known as SSPA, OJJDP selected 15 program sites across the country to implement a range of interventions for helping children and families cope with the effects of CEV. The 15 program sites varied in numerous ways, which are spelled out fully in a companion report, *National Evaluation of Safe Start Promising Approaches: Assessing Program Implementation* (Schultz et al., 2010). In short, the settings, populations served, intervention types, types of violence addressed, community partners, and program goals differed across sites. The RAND Corporation evaluated the performance of SSPA in each of the 15 program sites, in collaboration with the national evaluation team: OJJDP, the Safe Start Center, the Association for the Study and Development of Communities (ASDC), and the 15 program sites. The evaluation design involved three components: an outcomes evaluation; a process evaluation, including a program cost analysis; and an evaluation of program training efforts. This report presents the results of the outcomes evaluation.

Methods

The outcomes evaluations were designed to examine whether implementation of each Safe Start intervention was associated with individual-level changes in specific outcome domains. The evaluation utilized an intent-to-treat approach that is designed to inform policymakers about the types of outcomes that could be expected if a similar intervention were to be implemented in a similar setting. To prepare for the evaluation, the sites worked together with the national evaluation team to complete a "Green Light" process that developed the specific plans for the intervention and assured that the evaluation plan would align well with the intervention being offered and would be ethical and feasible to implement.

As a result of the Green Light process, a rigorous, controlled evaluation design was developed at each site, either with a randomized control group (wait list or alternative intervention) or a comparison group selected based on similar characteristics. Three sites had more than one study being conducted in their setting, as they delivered two different interventions to different groups of individuals. Overall, there were 18 separate evaluations of interventions within the 15 sites. Most sites utilized an experimental, randomized design (13 of 18), with RAND standardizing and monitoring the randomization procedures. Pre-intervention baseline data were collected on standardized, age-appropriate measures for all families enrolled in the studies. Longitudinal data on families were collected for within-site analysis of the impact of these programs on child outcomes at six, 12, 18, and 24 months post-enrollment. It should be noted that funding was relatively modest for designs of this type, requiring sites to leverage existing resources to the extent possible to maximize their ability to conduct the studies.

Measures for the national evaluation were chosen to document child and family outcomes in several domains: demographics, background and contextual, child and caregiver violence exposure, child behavior problems, child posttraumatic stress symptoms, child depressive symptoms, child social-emotional competence, parenting stress, caregiver-child relationship, and child school readiness/academic achievement. The 15 sites collected data with initial training and ongoing support from RAND and sent data to RAND for cleaning, scanning, and analysis.

Data analysis was performed for each site separately and included description of the baseline characteristics of families enrolled, description of the intervention services offered to these families, and mean responses on the outcome measures over time. The analysis of outcomes depended on the sample size, with more robust analyses and modeling possible with higher numbers of families in the samples.

Results

Descriptive analysis of the data collected confirmed the diversity of the interventions across the SSPA sites, with different types of families being served at the 15 sites. Across the sites, however, major impediments to the planned evaluations were the inability to recruit sufficient numbers of families for participation and difficulty retaining families for the follow-up assessments. Thus, none of the evaluations had adequate statistical power to detect whether the programs made an impact on participating children and families, and in some cases the samples were too low to complete exploratory analyses of changes within groups over time or differences between groups over time.

Within several sites, we noted promising improvements within the intervention groups over time. These include reductions in children's symptoms, improvement in resilience factors, and improvements in the parent-child relationship, depending on the site under study. In many cases, however, similar changes were noted in the control or comparison group, indicating that some outcomes may improve with the passage of time or by virtue of the general interventions received in the community.

Analyses of outcomes data in sites with marginally adequate statistical power to detect an intervention effect did not reveal any strong patterns of change in the outcomes in the intervention group as compared to controls. We present possible reasons for these findings, including both methodological and programmatic reasons, and discuss next steps relevant to each site in terms of both research and practice.

Detailed results for each site are included in the results appendixes and are summarized briefly here in the main report.

Conclusions

As focus on CEV has increased among researchers and public agencies, and its negative consequences on health, behavior, and development have become more evident, intervention programs have been developed to try to improve outcomes for these children. However, many of these programs lack evidence of efficacy or effectiveness on child-level outcomes, and the few that have been empirically evaluated have not been well tested in community settings. As such, the evaluations conducted as part of the SSPA are important, as they attempt to rigorously examine the effectiveness of such programs delivered in community settings, even with relatively modest funding levels. The level of rigor in evaluation attempted here is rarely seen in implementation projects that operate under real-world conditions.

The diversity of the SSPA programs under study is also noteworthy. Although the programs all focused on children exposed to violence, they varied considerably in terms of the type of intervention, the setting in which it was offered, and the group of children and families targeted for the intervention. All of the programs were able to successfully launch and provide some services to children and families exposed to violence, as reported in our report on SSPA implementation (Schultz et al., 2010).

Obstacles to the successful evaluation of these programs were numerous, and some of them were at least partially surmounted. These included developing measures that could assess the sensitive topic of violence exposure and examine outcomes across a range of ages, using advanced psychometric techniques to develop measures that would span a broader age range, working with multiple institutional review boards to assure confidentiality of the data collected and define the limits to confidentiality, and engaging community partners and families into the evaluation studies. Other obstacles were harder to overcome, including limits in funding, low uptake of the intervention services in some cases, and struggles with recruitment and/or retention. All of the challenges weakened the ability to draw firm conclusions from the data collected. Despite the limitations, these data will be useful in planning future research endeavors. The difficulties faced in conducting this outcome evaluation will also provide useful information about the types of challenges faced by families entering intervention services and the challenges in evaluating child outcomes in a variety of settings. Practitioners using interventions such as these, or in these types of settings, are advised to examine this report and the process evaluation report (Schultz et al., 2010) to understand the nature of problems they might encounter and families' willingness to accept or adhere to services.

In summary, while the outcomes evaluation overall produced no conclusive findings about the effectiveness of the interventions under study, the SSPA process evaluation identified many successes of the individual programs in implementing their program goals (Schultz et al., 2010). These successes included development of procedures for increased identification of children exposed to violence, improving communication and coordination among service providers, and establishment of new interagency and communitywide partnerships to address service gaps for children and their families. These improvements have value in their own right and should be considered as part of the legacy of the Safe Start Initiative.

Acknowledgments

This report would not have been possible without the many contributions of the Safe Start program staff and leadership at each of the 15 sites. We are extremely grateful for their generosity with their time and support during the data collection for this report and reviews of earlier drafts. Priya Sharma provided invaluable research assistance in the early phases of the project, and Alice Beckman supported the data cleaning phase of the project. Molly Scott and Al Crego provided programming assistance in the early part of the project. Scot Hickey set up the database and reporting functions for this project. We also thank Kristen Kracke and Jeffrey Gersh of OJJDP for their assistance and support with this effort. We also appreciate the important contributions of the RAND quality assurance peer reviewers, Beth Ann Griffin and Abigail Gewirtz. Their thoughtful comments helped improve the quality of this report.

Abbreviations

ASDC	Association for the Study and Development of Communities
ASQ	Ages and Stages Questionnaire
BERS-2	Behavior and Emotional Rating Scales—2
BITSEA	Brief Infant-Toddler Social and Emotional Assessment
BPI	Behavior Problems Index
CBCL	Child Behavior Checklist
CDI	Children's Depression Inventory
CEV	children's exposure to violence
CFI	comparative fit index
CPP	Child-Parent Psychotherapy
CPS	child protective services
EFA	exploratory factor analysis
ESI	Everyday Stressors Index
FDR	False Discovery Rate
FSS	Family Status Sheet
IMH	Infant Mental Health
IRB	institutional review board
IRT	item response theory
JVQ	Juvenile Victimization Questionnaire
LA FANS	Los Angeles Family and Neighborhood Survey
LONGSCAN	Longitudinal Studies of Child Abuse and Neglect
NCVS	National Victimization Crime Survey
NLSY	National Longitudinal Survey of Youth

NNFI	nonnormed fit index
NYS	National Youth Survey
OJJDP	Office of Juvenile Justice and Delinquency Prevention
PSI	Parenting Stress Index
PSI-SF	Parenting Stress Index—Short Form
PTSD	posttraumatic stress disorder
RAND HSPC	RAND Corporation Human Subjects Protection Committee
RCT	randomized controlled trial
RMSEA	root mean square error of approximation
RYDS	Rochester Youth Development Study
SSPA	Safe Start Promising Approaches
SSRS	Social Skills Rating System
TF-CBT	Trauma-Focused Cognitive Behavioral Therapy
TSCC	Trauma Symptom Checklist for Children
TSCYC	Trauma Symptom Checklist for Young Children
WJ-III	Woodcock-Johnson III scale
WLSM	Weighted Least Squares with adjusted Means

CHAPTER ONE

Introduction

Children's Exposure to Violence and Its Consequences

In recent years, the risk to children exposed to violence at home and in communities has gained wider recognition (Kracke and Hahn, 2008). A recent national study of the prevalence of children's exposure to violence (CEV) found that 61 percent of children had experienced or witnessed violence in the past year, with many experiencing multiple types of violence exposure (Finkelhor et al., 2009). Common sources of CEV are direct child maltreatment, witnessing domestic violence, and community and school violence. Child protective services agencies accepted 3.3 million referrals for neglect and abuse in 2008, and from these referrals, 772,000 children were found to be victims of abuse or neglect, representing a national rate of 10.3 per 1,000 children (Department of Health and Human Services, 2010). A high proportion of children are exposed to violence between adult intimate partners (Zinzow et al., 2009). Police data indicate that nearly half of domestic violence incidents include child witnesses (Fantuzzo et al., 2007; Fusco and Fantuzzo, 2009). Exposure to violence outside the home is also common. Our work in Los Angeles middle schools showed that 40 percent of children had been victimized in the community, and 63 percent had witnessed community violence in the prior year (Jaycox et al., 2002). Youth are also victims of violent crime at a rate of 26.5 per 1,000 (Baum, 2005).

The negative consequences of CEV include poor emotional, behavioral, and academic outcomes (see Margolin and Gordis [2000] for a review). A variety of psychiatric disorders and behavioral problems may result from direct or indirect CEV (Gilbert et al., 2009; Lansford et al., 2002; Morris, 2009). CEV has also been linked with posttraumatic stress disorder (PTSD; Berman et al., 1996; Breslau et al., 1997), depression (Kliewer et al., 1998), anxiety (Singer et al., 1995), and behavioral or developmental problems (Bell and Jenkins, 1993; Farrell and Bruce, 1997; Garbarino et al., 1992; Martinez and Richters, 1993). Symptoms that arise following CEV can impede school performance. Poorer school functioning and academic performance is more common in children exposed to community violence (Bowen and Bowen, 1999; Delaney-Black et al., 2002; Hurt et al., 2001; Schwartz and Gorman, 2003) or school violence (Grogger, 1997).

Resilience to Exposure to Violence

While CEV increases risk for negative outcomes, not all children exhibit problems. Even among children who have experienced multiple risks, approximately half will achieve developmental outcomes on pace with their peers who have not experienced similar disadvantage or exposure (Rutter, 2000). Understanding this "resilience" is a key to efforts to improve outcomes for children exposed to violence. Resilience is thought of as a dynamic process that influences an individual's capacity to adapt and function successfully despite experiencing risk or adversity. Resilience is not a trait or quality of an individual but is best thought of as a pattern of positive adaptation within the context of significant adversity (Luthar, Cicchetti, and Becker, 2000; Masten, 2001; Masten and Powell, 2003). Resilient children are those who, despite their increased risk, function *at least as well as* the average child who has not been exposed to adversity or a traumatic event (Luthar, Cicchetti, and Becker, 2000: Masten and Coatsworth, 1998).

Resilience is thought to operate through key protective factors at the individual, family, and community levels (Garmezy, 1985; Luthar, Cicchetti, and Becker, 2000; Werner, 1995). At the individual level, attributes such as intelligence, problem-solving skills, temperament, coping skills, and self-esteem can be protective against negative outcomes (Fergusson and Lynskey, 1996; Garmezy, Masten, and Tellegen, 1984; Masten, Best, and Garmezy, 1990; Rutter, 1986; Werner, 1995). At the family level, quality parent-child relationships and positive parenting skills are also predictors of resilience among at-risk children (Bradley et al., 1994; Cowen, Wyman, and Work, 1996; Gribble et al., 1993). At the community level, schools, churches, and social service organizations can provide support to children exposed to violence (Masten and Powell, 2003; Rak and Patterson, 1996). Social networks play an essential role in providing children with these key protective factors by helping to mitigate against risk-taking behavior (Fitzpatrick, 1997; Loury, 1977).

Promising Practices to Improve Outcomes for Children Exposed to Violence

Given the range of deleterious outcomes experienced by children exposed to violence, effective prevention and intervention programs are clearly needed. Such programs can focus on reducing the occurrence of additional violence exposure, reducing the negative impacts on children, enhancing resilience factors, or a combination of these. Such efforts can take place in a variety of settings. For instance, the protection of children has largely become the function of child protective services (CPS) agencies that receive referrals, investigate, and respond to allegations of maltreatment and exposure to domestic violence. Clinical social workers in these agencies assess child victims, make recommendations for treatment and placement, and refer to law enforcement for criminal investigation (Schene, 1998). CPS agencies may also provide referrals to the caregivers for parenting classes, housing assistance, substance abuse treatment, day care, and counseling. Other agencies also play a critical role. Juvenile and family courts conduct hearings on allegations of abuse and exposure to violence and decide whether a child should be removed from home. Law enforcement agencies investigate allegations and make arrests, while criminal courts become involved in cases referred for prosecution. Coordination and integration of these efforts is critical to ensuring positive outcomes for children. Some promising practices, such as the Greenbook Initiative, focus on developing relationships across agencies to ensure substantive collaboration among law enforcement, child welfare, domestic violence, courts, and other agencies that encounter children exposed to direct and/or indirect violence (Schechter and Edleson, 1999).

Within the mental health care system that often receives referrals for CEV, there is increasing emphasis on delivery of evidence-based care to these children. Examples include prevention programs that promote safe, stable, and nurturing families, such as the Nurse-Family Partnership or Triple P—Positive Parenting Program, which have been demonstrated to improve children's chances of future social and psychological well-being (Mercy and Saul, 2009; Prinz et al., 2009). Targeted school-based prevention programs that focus on symptomatic children who have been exposed to violence have also demonstrated effectiveness (see Jaycox, Stein, and Amaya-Jackson [2008] for a full review). Finally, treatment options exist for young children (such as Child-Parent Psychotherapy [CPP]; Lieberman and Van Horn, 2005) or for specific symptoms, like PTSD (such as Trauma-Focused Cognitive Behavioral Therapy [TF-CBT]; Cohen, Mannarino, and Deblinger, 2006), with some suggestion of additive benefits in interventions focusing on both parent and child exposure to violence at home (Rivett, Howarth, and Harold, 2006).

Despite some progress toward identifying evidence-based programs and practices, the programs to date are limited in their reach (e.g., age range, setting, or target symptoms) and, for the most part, have not been well tested in community settings. Demonstration projects have rarely moved beyond description to rigorously test interventions to evaluate their impact. Thus, community practitioners have little research from which to draw when attempting to address the needs of the multiply stressed and trauma-exposed families with whom they work. Research that tests promising and proven programs, as well as new programs in real-world settings, is a critical need.

The Safe Start Initiative

The dual need to develop better programs and practices for children exposed to violence—and to prove that they can work in community settings—was the impetus for the Safe Start Initiative. The Office of Juvenile Justice and Delinquency Prevention (OJJDP) launched the Safe Start Initiative in 2000. Safe Start is a community-based initiative focused on developing, fielding, and evaluating interventions to prevent and reduce the impact of CEV. It consists of four phases:

- **Phase One:** Phase One focused on expanding the system of care for children exposed to violence by conducting demonstration projects. Completed in 2006, this phase involved demonstrations of various innovative, promising practices in the system of care for children who have been exposed to violence.
- **Phase Two:** Building on Phase One, this phase was intended to implement and evaluate promising and evidence-based programs in community settings to identify how well programs worked in reducing and preventing the harmful effects of CEV. This phase is the subject of this report.
- **Phase Three:** The aim of this phase will be to build a knowledge base of effective interventions in the field of CEV.
- **Phase Four:** The goal of this phase will be to "seed" on a national scale the effective strategies identified in the earlier phases.

Overview of 15 Phase Two Safe Start Sites

This report focuses on Phase Two of the Safe Start program. For this phase, known as Safe Start Promising Approaches (SSPA), OJJDP selected 15 program sites across the country to implement a range of interventions for helping children and families cope with the effects of CEV.

Program sites were located in the following 15 communities:

- Bronx, New York
- Broward County, Florida
- Chelsea, Massachusetts
- Dallas, Texas
- Dayton, Ohio
- Erie, Pennsylvania
- Kalamazoo, Michigan
- Miami, Florida
- Multnomah County, Oregon
- Oakland, California
- Providence, Rhode Island
- San Diego County, California
- San Mateo County, California
- Toledo, Ohio
- Washington Heights/Inwood, New York.

The program sites varied in numerous ways (see Schultz et al. [2010] for a full description of each program design and its implementation). In brief, the sites focused on addressing multiple types of violence exposure and offered different interventions for such exposure, including variations in target ages and age-appropriate practices. The 15 program sites also varied in size, location, and population characteristics. Each of the communities had identified barriers to services for children exposed to violence and viewed SSPA as an opportunity to increase capacity, coordinate services, and address gaps in the array of services in the community. The SSPA programs were situated locally within different kinds of lead agencies or organizations, including health clinics or hospitals, human services agencies, organizational units within universities, domestic violence or child maltreatment services agencies, and county-level government offices. In developing their programs, the lead agencies partnered with the specific agencies in their community that routinely encounter children who have been exposed to violence, including law enforcement agencies, child protective services agencies, human services agencies, behavioral health organizations, and other community nonprofit agencies. The programs varied in their source of referrals, including the clinic or hospital system, child welfare system, domestic violence shelters, human services agencies, Head Start, or a combination of the above.

The 15 Safe Start programs comprised a range of intervention components. All included a therapeutic component; about two-thirds focused on dyadic therapy (therapy that includes the child and a parent or caregiver) or family therapy, while the rest used individual or group therapy approaches. In some cases, the modality varied by age, with dyadic or family therapy for younger children and group therapy for older children. Many of the sites also offered case management and/or established or enhanced interagency service coordination for families.

Some of the sites had other intervention components, such as family or child-level advocacy, parent/caregiver groups, or other services (e.g., multidisciplinary evaluation of family needs, an in-home safety assessment, etc.). The intervention setting also varied, with interventions offered in families' homes, clinics, shelters, child centers, or Head Start classrooms. The interventions varied in length from three months to more than one year. See Schultz et al. (2010) for a detailed description of each program.

At all of the sites, the interventions were conducted in the context of a rigorous evaluation, as required by OJJDP, although the evaluation at the Toledo, Ohio, site was discontinued near the end of the project. The RAND Corporation was selected to serve as the evaluator after the program sites and intervention models had been selected by OJJDP. RAND researchers evaluated the programs in collaboration with a national evaluation team that comprised OJJDP, the Safe Start Center, the Association for the Study and Development of Communities (ASDC), and the 15 program sites. The evaluation design involved three components: a process evaluation, which included a cost analysis; an evaluation of training; and an outcomes evaluation. The process evaluation and training evaluation can be found in Schultz et al. (2010). The outcomes evaluation is the subject of the present report.

Outcome Evaluation Overview

The outcome evaluation was designed to examine whether interventions are associated with individual-level changes in specific outcome domains at a particular site. For the evaluation, a rigorous, controlled evaluation design was developed at each site, either with a randomized control group (wait list or alternative intervention) or a comparison group selected based on similar characteristics. A listing of the characteristics of each site, along with the evaluation design employed, can be seen in Table 1.1.

The evaluation utilized an intent-to-treat approach designed to inform policymakers about the types of outcomes that could be expected if a similar program were to be implemented in a similar setting. This approach includes all of those who are offered participation in a program, regardless of how much of the program they actually participate in, and thus shows the potential impact of a program on children at a community level. This differs from a completer analysis approach, in which only those who successfully complete treatment are included, answering the question of how well a program works for those that participate fully. Longitudinal data on families were collected for within-site analysis of the impact of these programs on child outcomes at six, 12, 18, and 24 months post-enrollment. The data included demographics, violence exposure, outcomes (PTSD symptoms, depressive symptoms, behavior problems, parenting stress), and resilience data at the child level.

Funding for the studies was relatively modest. Sites received $210,000 per year for their project (including both direct and indirect costs) and were allowed to spend no more than $10,000 per year on data collection for families in the intervention condition. The RAND Corporation received a larger grant to conduct the evaluation and to support data collection for families in the control or comparison condition. RAND subcontracted to the sites a range of $10,300 to $19,400 in the first year and from $6,000 to $80,000 in subsequent years to cover costs of control group data collection, as well as to augment data collection for the intervention families. This level of funding is modest compared with clinical trials, despite the large

Table 1.1
Program Site Characteristics and Evaluation Designs

Site and Lead Agency/ Organization	Intervention Components	Target Population	Planned Evaluation Design
The Bronx, N.Y.: St. Barnabas Hospital's Children's Advocacy Center	Medical Home for Children Exposed to Violence, including multidisciplinary assessment, CPP, and case management	Children ages 0–6 who have been exposed to, have experienced, or have witnessed family or community violence	Randomized controlled trial comparing intervention with enhanced usual care
Broward County, Fla.: Institute for Family Centered Services, Inc.	Family-Centered Treatment®	Children ages 0–8 who have been exposed to all types of violence, with a focus on exposure to domestic violence	Randomized controlled trial comparing intervention with a 6-month wait-list control group
Chelsea, Mass.: Massachusetts General Hospital's Chelsea Health Care Center	Group therapy, home visits, and case coordination	Children ages 0–17 who have been exposed to violence	Quasi-experimental comparison of patients at intervention clinic compared with patients at control clinic
Dallas, Tex.: Department of Psychology, Southern Methodist University	Project Support, including therapy, case management, and child mentorship	Children ages 3–9 exiting domestic violence shelters with their mothers who have been exposed to domestic violence	Randomized controlled trial comparing intervention with enhanced usual care
Dayton, Ohio: Artemis Center for Alternatives to Domestic Violence	CPP and case management/coordination	Children ages 0–5 who have been exposed to domestic violence	Randomized controlled trial comparing intervention with usual care
Erie, Pa.: Children's Advocacy Center of Erie County	Individualized therapy, case coordination, and parent education groups	Children ages 0–12 who have been physically or sexually abused, have witnessed domestic violence, have been a victim of any violent crime, or have witnessed a violent crime	Randomized controlled trial comparing intervention with usual care
Kalamazoo, Mich.: Child Trauma Assessment Center, Western Michigan University	Head Start School Intervention Project, teacher training, and parent training program	Children ages 3–5 who have been exposed to violence	Cluster randomized controlled trial comparing intervention with usual care, with randomization at the classroom level
Miami, Fla.: Linda Ray Center, Department of Psychology, University of Miami	PREVENT assessment, Infant Mental Health (IMH)—CPP for children from 6 months to 5 years old, Heroes group therapy, and enhanced case management for children ages 6 through 12	Children ages 0–12 residing in specific shelters who have been exposed to domestic violence, have been exposed to community violence, and/or have experienced abuse or neglect; or court-referred children for clinic-based treatment	Quasi-experimental comparison of participants at intervention shelters compared with participants at control shelters, augmented with a randomized controlled trial comparing intervention with a six-month wait-list control group
Multnomah County, Ore.: Multnomah County Domestic Violence Coordinator's Office	Domestic violence advocacy, CPP, and case coordination and consultation	Children ages 0–6 within a county child welfare population who have been exposed to domestic violence	Quasi-experimental comparison of participants at an intervention child welfare agency compared with participants at a control child welfare agency

Table 1.1—Continued

Site and Lead Agency/ Organization	Intervention Components	Target Population	Planned Evaluation Design
Oakland, Calif.: Safe Passages	Case management integrated with dyadic caregiver/child psychotherapy	Children ages 0–5 who have been exposed to domestic violence, have been exposed to community violence, and/or have experienced abuse or neglect	Randomized controlled trial comparing intervention with usual care.
Providence, R.I.: Family Service of Rhode Island (FSRI)	Tier 1: Crisis intervention	Children ages 0–18 who have been exposed to domestic or community violence	Not evaluated
	Tier 2: Case management		Quasi-experimental comparison of participants at an intervention domestic violence shelter compared with participants at a control shelter
	Tier 3: CPP and case management		Randomized controlled trial comparing intervention with usual care
San Diego, Calif.: Office of Violence Prevention, San Diego County Health and Human Services Agency	Trauma-Focused Cognitive-Behavioral Therapy, child advocacy, and case coordination	Children ages 3–12 within a county child welfare population who have been exposed to domestic violence	Randomized controlled trial comparing intervention with usual care
San Mateo, Calif.: Edgewood Center for Children and Families	CPP	Children ages 0–7 in kinship care who have been exposed to domestic violence, have been exposed to community violence, and/or have experienced abuse or neglect	Randomized controlled trial comparing intervention with usual care
Toledo, Ohio Toledo Children's Hospital's Cullen Center[a]	CPP	Children ages 0–5 who have been exposed to domestic violence	Randomized controlled trial comparing intervention with usual care
Washington Heights/ Inwood, N.Y.: New York Presbyterian Hospital's Ambulatory Care Network	CPP for children ages 0–5, Kids' Club and Reflective Parent Group for children ages 6–12.	Children ages 0–12 who have been exposed to domestic violence	Randomized controlled trial comparing intervention with a six-month wait-list control group

NOTE: CPP = Child-Parent Psychotherapy.

[a] The evaluation at the Toledo, Ohio, site was discontinued near the end of the project, although services continued. Data gathered are presented in the results appendixes, but Toledo is not discussed in the rest of this report.

challenges of conducting effectiveness trials in real-world settings, and should be noted when examining the results of this report.

In the rest of this report, we report on the methods used in these studies (planning and start-up activities, measures, data collection) and present a short overview of results. The detailed results for each site can be found in the results appendixes (http://www.rand.org/pubs/technical_reports/TR991-1.html). We then discuss the implications of these results and recommendations for next steps.

CHAPTER TWO

Site Start-Up and Planning

The Green Light Process

Prior to using program funds, hiring staff, or conducting other implementation activities, each site participated in the Green Light process. (This process and resulting changes in each site are more fully described in our companion report, Schultz et al. [2010]). The purpose of the process was to make sure that sites were (1) ready to start implementation and (2) ready to be part of the evaluation. No formal evaluation data were collected until after the Green Light process was completed.

This process consisted of a review by the national evaluation team of a checklist of criteria. The checklist was developed by RAND researchers in consultation with the national evaluation team to ensure that each site had the key components in place for implementation of its program and for participation in the national evaluation. As shown in Table 2.1, the Green Light criteria included 28 items focusing on five areas: (1) program design, (2) control/comparison groups, (3) data collection, (4) RAND and local Institutional Review Board (IRB) approval, and (5) stakeholder agreements. Each site was asked to document its specific capabilities and plans in each area through an iterative process with the national evaluation team, culminating in receipt of Green Light approval from OJJDP and RAND for each site to begin implementation and evaluation activities.

The process also provided an opportunity for sites to receive technical assistance in areas of need related to their intervention or evaluation, which in some cases resulted in changes to sites' original implementation plans. For some sites, the evaluation component was completely redesigned from what the site had proposed in its original request for funding to OJJDP. Some project leaders needed extensive guidance regarding the data collection and evaluation issues. The Green Light process provided an opportunity to explain the research component, randomization procedures (where applicable), and IRB requirements and approvals that were necessary to participate in a research project.

In some cases, the programs needed to train their own staff and educate their community partners on the overall initiative, the specific program plans, and the importance of the associated research. Some sites took additional time (up to four months) between the Green Light date and their actual start date to begin implementation. Six of the sites received more-intensive technical assistance during the Green Light process to help complete the checklist. The technical assistance was provided by the national evaluation team and involved conference calls, in-person meetings, and review of materials, as necessary. The focus of technical assistance included the program design, implementation strategy, and target population.

Table 2.1
Green Light Process Checklist

Category	Item
Program Design	Intervention is theory- and evidence-based and appropriate to the defined target population.
	Project logic model reflects theory base for implementation.
	Case flow is projected for both the intervention and comparison/control groups.
	Site has clearly defined • target population • key elements of the intervention that distinguish it from usual services • referral sources to the program • entrance and inclusion/exclusion criteria • starting point of the intervention • criteria for ending the intervention • criteria for when to count a case as a "dropout."
	Staff has been trained in the intervention.
	Where applicable, sites have a plan for • determining the duration for different elements of the intervention • determining how cases will be assigned to each level or type of intervention.
Control/Comparison Group	Relationships are established that ensure referrals into both intervention and comparison/control groups.
	Sites can create a control group within the program (e.g., by randomizing) that is • feasible (no "spillover" of intervention services to the control group) • ethical (all families receive some services, stakeholder buy-in).
	If a control group is not feasible, a site has access to a comparison group that is • not exposed to the key elements of the program • identified in the same way as the intervention group • similar to the intervention group • feasible (no "spillover" of services, selected before services begin).
Data Collection	A data collection person is identified who can oversee data collection for all participants (both comparison/control and intervention).
	Training has been received from RAND on data collection and submission procedures.
IRB Approval: RAND and Local	The IRB application • defines RAND's role • contains RAND's consent language.
	The local IRB approval has been obtained and sent to RAND.
Stakeholder Agreement	All partners have agreed to participate in • finalized service delivery/implementation plans • evaluation plans, including plans for comparison/control group and data collection.

In sum, the Green Light process enabled the sites and OJJDP to define the interventions in more detail, coordinate the intervention design with the evaluation, receive technical assistance in areas of need, and ensure readiness for implementation and evaluation. This allowed the sites to be fully ready to implement their programs and evaluation activities at the start of the evaluation. Sites were not permitted by OJJDP to make substantial changes to their programs during the evaluation, although small changes were approved for many sites to accommodate unexpected issues (e.g., expansion of the age range, inclusion of an additional referral source, and the like). Thus, the interventions were relatively stable during the evaluation period (see Schultz et al. [2010]).

Human Subjects Protections

Consideration of research ethics and protection of human participants were important aspects of planning, as well as of the ongoing implementation of the programs and the evaluation. Thirteen of the 15 sites utilized their own IRBs for review and monitoring of the evaluation, in addition to obtaining a secondary review from the RAND Corporation Human Subjects Protection Committee (RAND HSPC). The remaining two sites did not have IRBs of their own and utilized the RAND HSPC for the entire approval and monitoring process.

At the beginning of the project, the RAND HSPC worked with the evaluation team to develop language about the national evaluation and RAND's role in data collection that could be incorporated into each site's participant consent forms and materials. Sites were allowed to modify the language if they wished, or they could use it as written when they submitted materials to their own IRBs.

Protocols and requirements at each site differed, with unique issues and concerns arising at different institutions. For instance, hospital-based programs needed to work through issues related to patient privacy (e.g., the Health Insurance Portability and Accountability Act [HIPAA]), and sites working with individuals in the child welfare system or with court-referred families needed to work through issues related to voluntariness of the research to ensure that no families felt pressured to participate. Sites also had to work through processes for identifying legal guardians (when separate from primary caregivers) and obtaining consent for participation. Sites were required to report incidents during the study both to their local IRB and to the RAND HSPC to ensure that both committees were apprised of issues during the study and able to make recommendations for remediation or changes in protocol.

CHAPTER THREE

Measures

To assess outcomes at each site, we used a set of measures that captured background and contextual factors, as well as a broad array of outcomes, including PTSD symptoms, depressive symptoms, behavior/conduct problems, social-emotional competence, caregiver-child relationship, school readiness/performance, and violence exposure.

As described in the introduction of this report and in our summary of the process evaluation (Schultz et al., 2010), the 15 Safe Start sites differed in intervention, setting, and target population. Thus, choosing measures that could be used across all 15 sites was challenging. Our goal was to identify measures meeting the following criteria:

- The measure could be administered by lay interviewers rather than by highly trained clinicians, in order to fit into budgetary and staffing constraints.
- The measure had been widely accepted and widely used in the field, which maximizes credibility to the sites and to the ultimate audience of the results of the evaluation.
- The measure or subscale of a measure adhered closely to the outcome domains specified by the Safe Start goals.
- The measure could be used with a broad age range so that as many children as possible could be evaluated on each measure and to minimize the number of different measures needed within a site.
- To minimize burden on participants, brevity was considered when selecting a measure. Our goal was to develop an assessment packet with measures that would take less than one hour to complete.
- Measures that had demonstrated sensitivity to change in the child as demonstrated in prior intervention studies were prioritized because of the importance of being able to detect changes in the evaluation.
- A Spanish-language version of the measure was available, or translation was feasible.

Restricting the evaluation to include Spanish speakers as the only non-English group was not ideal. Several sites, particularly Oakland, were interested in including other groups in the evaluated services. Because of the multiple complications introduced by producing consistent and reliable translations of other languages, it was simply not feasible to expand the evaluation further.

When we had difficulty finding measures that could be used across a broad age range, we planned overlap in administration of the measures we did locate. For instance, if we had one measure valid for children ages 1–3 and another measure on the same construct that was valid for children ages 3–10, we planned to have the 3-year-olds complete both measures. This allowed us to conduct psychometric work to combine the measures for use across the entire 1–10 age range, which is discussed in more detail below.

With such a broad age range, some aspects of child functioning could be reported with more validity by a caregiver, whereas other aspects could be reported with more validity by the child. Thus, caregivers completed most of the measures for young children. Caregivers completed fewer measures for older children because older children were invited to complete self-report measures. Measures for caregivers and children (ages 3 and up) were assembled into two batteries: a caregiver assessment battery and a child assessment battery. A Family Status Sheet (FSS), which documented services received and current status of the family's engagement with services, was also completed for all families at each assessment point.

To appropriately capture outcomes for the different age groups at each of the 15 different intervention sites, two accommodations were made:

1. Sites received assessment batteries containing only the instruments appropriate for the ages of participating children.
2. While sites collected all age-appropriate measures in the assessment batteries, they were invited to prioritize these measures, for purposes of outcome evaluation analysis, according to the measures they expected to be most impacted by their intervention.

Overall, the study captured the following eight outcome domains:

- Background and Contextual Factors
- PTSD Symptoms
- Depressive Symptoms
- Behavior/Conduct Problems
- Social-Emotional Competence
- Caregiver-Child Relationship
- School Readiness/Performance
- Violence Exposure.

The next two sections describe each domain in more detail and the measures used to capture them, first for the caregiver assessment battery and then for the child assessment battery. We then provide an overview of the entire assessment across both caregivers and children. Following that section, we describe the measures within domains in more detail.

In our descriptions of each measure, we included the following information: (1) the number of items, (2) the age(s) for whom the measure is appropriate, (3) the type of questions asked and response scales, (4) scoring and interpretation of the questions, (5) a brief explanation about why the measure was selected (over other similar measures) and any modifications made to the measure, (6) a summary of the measure's reliability and validity, and (7) the Cronbach's alpha, a measure of internal consistency of the measure, from the Safe Start sample. If we only used a subset of scales from the measure, an explanation of why we did not use the other scales in the measure was also included in the description. Because the same measures may have been used across multiple domains and by both children and caregivers, we describe the measure in detail *only* the first time it is mentioned. Information on Spanish-language translations of each measure can be found at the end of this chapter.

Measures are named in this report so that a higher score indicates more of the named construct. That is, a higher score on a measure of social-emotional competence means more competence, and a higher score on a measure of PTSD symptoms means more symptoms.

Caregiver Assessment Battery

Caregivers completed a battery of instruments that comprised between 95 and 249 items, depending on the age of the child. This battery took between 38 and 86 minutes to complete. Table 3.1 shows the variations in caregiver measures and the number of items by the age of the participating child. Details of the administration of the caregiver assessment battery are described in the data collection section of this report.

Child Assessment Battery

Children ages three and older were assessed. The assessment battery comprised between 36 to 165 items, depending on the age of the child. The child assessment battery also varied by the age of the child. Table 3.2 shows the child assessment battery by the age of the child. Details of the administration of the child assessment battery are described in the data collection section of this report.

Assessment Strategy of Domains by Caregivers and Children

Across caregivers and children, the eight outcome domains were covered as shown in Table 3.3. Additional details on the specific topic areas are included in the next section under the corresponding domain.

Background and Contextual Factors

Three measures were completed by caregivers to capture background and context.

Caregiver Report of Demographics and Service Use. Basic demographics of the caregiver, such as age, education, employment status, income, primary language, citizenship status, race/ethnicity, and marital status, were collected using the Caregiver Demographics and Service Use instrument, which was adapted from materials used in the Longitudinal Studies of Child Abuse and Neglect (LONGSCAN study; LONGSCAN, 2010), a consortium of longitudinal research studies assessing the etiology and impact of child maltreatment. This instrument also collects information on the caregiver's physical health, emotional problems, and support or assistance received. The instrument has a total of 15 items.

Caregiver Report of Child Demographics and Service Use. Basic demographics of the child, such as age, gender, race/ethnicity, primary language, citizenship status, and primary caregiver, were collected using the Child Demographics and Service Use instrument, which was adapted from materials used in the LONGSCAN study. The section on service use collects information on the child's physical health, medical problems, and behavioral, emotional, or school problems. The instrument has a total of 18 items.

Table 3.1
Number of Items in Caregiver Assessment Battery by Age of Child

Domain	Measure	<1	1–2	3	4–5	6–10	11–12	Teen
Background and Contextual Factors	Child Demographics and Service Use	18	18	18	18	18	18	18
	Caregiver Demographics and Service Use	15	15	15	15	15	15	15
	Everyday Stressors Index	20	20	20	20	20	20	20
PTSD Symptoms	Trauma Symptom Checklist for Young Children (PTSD Scale)	—	—	27	27	27	—	—
Behavior/ Conduct Problems	Brief Infant–Toddler Social and Emotional Assessment (Problem Scale)	—	31	31	—	—	—	—
	Behavior Problem Index (Externalizing Scale)	—	—	16	16	16	16	16
	Behavior Problem Index (Internalizing Scale)	—	—	16	16	16	16	16
Social-Emotional Competence	Ages and Stages Questionnaire	6	6	—	—	—	—	—
	Brief Infant–Toddler Social and Emotional Assessment (Social-Emotional Competence Scale)	—	11	11	—	—	—	—
	Social Skills Rating System 3–5: Cooperation, Assertion, and Self-Control	—	—	30	30	—	—	—
	Behavior and Emotional Rating Scales—2 (BERS-2; School Functioning and Affective Strengths Scales)	—	—	—	—	17	17	—
	Social Skills Rating System 6–12: Cooperation, Assertion, and Self-Control	—	—	—	—	30	30	—
Caregiver-Child Relationship	BERS-2 (Family Involvement Scale)	—	—	—	—	9	9	—
	Parenting Stress Index—Short Form	36	36	36	36	36	36	—
Violence Exposure	Juvenile Victimization Questionnaire	19	19	19	19	19	19	—
	Caregiver Victimization Questionnaire	10	10	10	10	10	10	10
Total		124	166	249	207	233	206	95

Caregiver Report of Everyday Stressors. To assess problems faced in everyday life, we used the Everyday Stressors Index (ESI) from the LONGSCAN study, which included 20 items from the 117-item Daily Hassles Scale developed by Kanner and colleagues (Hall, 1983). The 20 items tap five problem areas: role overload, financial concerns, parenting worries, employment problems, and interpersonal conflict. Caregivers are asked to rate the extent to which each problem bothered them "from day to day" (4 = bothered a great deal, 3 = somewhat

Table 3.2
Number of Items in Child Assessment Battery by Age of Child

Domain	Measure	3–7	8–10	11–12	Teen
PTSD Symptoms	TSCC (PTSD Scale)	—	10	10	10
Depressive Symptoms	Child Depression Inventory	—	26	26	26
Behavior/Conduct Problems	Delinquency Behavior (modified from three measures)	—	—	18	18
Social-Emotional Competence	Social Skills Rating System 13–18: Cooperation, Assertion, and Self-Control	—	—	—	30
	BERS-2 (School Functioning and Affective Strengths Scales)	—	—	17	17
Caregiver-Child Relationship	BERS-2 (Family Involvement Scale)	—	—	9	9
School Readiness/Performance	Woodcock-Johnson III[a]	36	36	36	36
Violence Exposure	Juvenile Victimization Questionnaire	—	—	19	19
Total		**36**	**72**	**135**	**165**

[a] The number of items for the Woodcock-Johnson III scale varies, but the total scale takes 9–21 minutes to complete. On average we found that children completed 36 items, so we have used that data to help estimate the total number of items per assessment battery by the age of the child.

NOTE: TSCC = Trauma Symptom Checklist for Children.

bothered, 2 = a little bothered, and 1 = not at all bothered). Internal consistency for the ESI was reported as high, with a Cronbach's alpha of 0.83 (Hall, Williams, and Greenberg, 1985). Construct validity of the ESI was supported by discrimination of everyday stressors from measures of maternal depression and psychosomatic symptoms using factor analytic procedures (Hall, 1983). Also, Hall and Farel (1988) reported that scores on the ESI were positively and significantly associated with depressive symptoms (as measured by the Center for Epidemiological Studies—Depression scale) and psychosomatic symptoms (as measured by the Health Opinion Survey), among a sample of unmarried mothers.

We conducted exploratory and confirmatory factor analyses on the 20 items in the ESI using data from 1,517 caregivers assessed at baseline. Items were modeled as categorical using the Mplus software, and the Weighted Least Squares with adjusted Means (WLSM) estimator was used (Muthen and Muthen, 1998–2004). The analysis identified a two-factor solution that was easily interpretable and resulted in high internal consistency within each factor. Namely, from the 20 items, we created a score for resource problems based on seven items (Cronbach's alpha = 0.81) and for personal/family problems based on 13 items (Cronbach's alpha = 0.80) for use in our evaluation. The resource problem scale included items tapping issues related to poverty, such as owing money or getting credit, not having enough money for basic necessities, problems with housing, and the like. The personal/family problem scale tapped the remaining items having to do with concerns about health, concerns about children, disagreements with others, and having too many responsibilities. We computed a total score for each subscale on this measure that can range from 0 to 28 for the resource problems subscale and from 0 to 52 for the personal/family problems subscale, with a higher score indicating more-severe problems.

Table 3.3
Assessment Strategy by Respondent, Age, and Specific Topic Areas Within Domain

Domain	Respondent	Specific Topic Area	Age Range
Background and Contextual Factors	Caregiver	Caregiver Demographics and Service Use	0–18
	Caregiver	Child Demographics and Service Use	0–18
	Caregiver	Everyday Stressors	0–18
PTSD Symptoms	Caregiver	Child PTSD Symptoms	3–10
	Child	Child PTSD Symptoms	8–18
Depressive Symptoms	Child	Child Depressive Symptoms	8–18
Behavior/Conduct Problems	Caregiver	Child Behavior Problems	1–18
	Child	Delinquency	11–18
Social-Emotional Competence	Caregiver	Child Personal-Social Competence	0–2
	Caregiver	Child Self-Control and Child Assertion	1–12
	Caregiver	Child Cooperation	3–12
	Child	Child Social Skills: Cooperation, Assertion, Self-Control	13–18
	Caregiver	Child Affective Strengths and School Functioning	6–12
	Child	Child Affective Strengths and School Functioning	11–18
Caregiver-Child Relationship	Caregiver	Parenting Stress	0–11
	Caregiver	Family Involvement	6–12
	Child	Family Involvement	11–18
School Readiness/Performance	Child	Child Achievement: Word Identification, Passage Comprehension, Applied Problems	3–18
Violence Exposure	Caregiver	Juvenile Victimization	0–12
	Caregiver	Caregiver Victimization	0–18
	Child	Juvenile Victimization	11–18

PTSD Symptoms

We used two measures to assess child PTSD symptoms, one reported by caregivers for young children, and the second reported by children themselves.

Caregiver Report of Child PTSD Symptoms. To assess caregivers' perceptions of PTSD symptoms in younger children, ages 3 to 10, we used the Trauma Symptom Checklist for Young Children (TSCYC; Briere et al., 2001). This measure includes subscales for PTSD, depression, and anxiety. With permission from the developers, we used only the PTSD subscale. The TSCYC PTSD scale includes 27 items that tap things the child does, feels, or experiences (e.g., bad dreams or nightmares, being bothered by memories of something that happened to him or her) and asks caregivers to rate the frequency of these events in the last month (4 = very often, 3 = often, 2 = sometimes, and 1 = not at all).

In prior research, the TSCYC has been shown to have good internal consistency, with a Cronbach's alpha of 0.87 (Briere et al., 2001). In the present study, the Cronbach's alpha was 0.93. Additionally, discriminant, predictive, and construct validity have been demonstrated for the TSCYC in multiple samples and studies (Briere et al., 2001; Pollio, Glover-Orr, and Wherry, 2008). We computed a total score for this measure that can range from 27 to 108, with a higher score indicating more PTSD symptoms. In addition, we used categories of symptoms based on norms by age and gender to describe the sample as having normal, borderline, or significant symptoms.

Child Self-Report of PTSD Symptoms. To assess children's own perception of PTSD symptoms, we used the Trauma Symptom Checklist for Children (TSCC; Briere, 1996) among children ages 8 to 18. This measure includes subscales for PTSD, depression, and anxiety. With permission from the developers, we used only the PTSD subscale. The TSCC PTSD scale contains ten items that tap feelings, thoughts, and behavior (e.g., bad dreams or nightmares, remembering scary things) by having children rate the frequency with which they experience each (3 = almost all the time, 2 = lots of times, 1 = sometimes, 0 = never). The PTSD scale has been shown in prior research to have good internal consistency, with a Cronbach's alpha of 0.82 (Briere, 1996), and in this project the Cronbach's alpha was 0.80. One study found that the TSCC displays good sensitivity to the effects of therapy for abused children (Lanktree and Briere, 1995). We compute a total score for this measure that can range from 0 to 30, with a higher score indicating more PTSD symptoms. In addition, we used categories of symptoms based on norms by age and gender to describe the sample as having normal, borderline, or significant symptoms.

Depressive Symptoms

To assess depressive symptoms in children age 8 and older, we selected one self-report instrument.

Self-Report of Child Depressive Symptoms. The Children's Depression Inventory (CDI; Kovacs, 1981) is a 26-item measure that assesses children's cognitive, affective, and behavioral depressive symptoms and is used for children 8 to 18 years of age. We excluded one item on suicidal ideation/intent. The child is given three statements and asked to pick the one that best describes her or him in the past two weeks (e.g., I am sad once in a while, I am sad many times, I am sad all the time). Each item is scored on a 0–2 scale, with the more-extreme distress item rated as a 2. The CDI has been proven to be a reliable and valid test, with Cronbach's alphas ranging from 0.80 to 0.88, a sensitivity of 80 percent, and a specificity of 84 percent (Kovacs, 2003). Validity has also been demonstrated, with correlates in the expected direction between the CDI and measures of related constructs, e.g. self-esteem, negative attributions, and hopelessness (Kendall, Cantwell, and Kazdin, 1989). In the current study, the Cronbach's alpha was 0.88. Total scores were derived on this scale ranging from 0 to 52, with a higher score indicating more depressive symptoms.

Behavior/Conduct Problems

To assess internalizing and externalizing behavior problems and delinquency, we used several measures and combined them using advanced psychometric techniques to develop a score that could be used across a broader age range. For sites that did not span the age range and worked only with children age 3 or older, we used the original measure, as described in the next section.

Caregiver Report of Child Behavioral Problems. Two measures were used to develop a score for total behavior problems. To assess conduct problems for children between the ages of 1 and 3, we used the Brief Infant-Toddler Social and Emotional Assessment (BITSEA; Briggs-Gowan and Carter, 2002). On this measure, caregivers report 31 items related to behavioral problems (e.g., seems nervous, tense, or fearful; is restless and can't sit still) on a three-point scale (1 = not true or rarely, 2 = somewhat true or sometimes, and 3 = very true or often). This measure has been shown to have good reliability and validity, with BITSEA problems correlating highly with concurrent evaluator problem ratings and predicting problem scores one year later (Briggs-Gowan et al., 2004). To assess behavior/conduct problems for ages 3–18, we used the Behavior Problems Index (BPI; Peterson and Zill, 1986) along with four additional items that had been used as part of the National Longitudinal Survey of Youth (NLSY). In this scale, the caregiver is asked to assess the validity (2 = often true, 1 = sometimes true, and 0 = not true) of statements about the child's behavior in the past month (e.g., he/she has been too fearful or anxious, he/she has argued too much). The scale has been demonstrated to have good internal consistency for each of its components (for externalizing problems, the Cronbach's alpha was 0.86; for internalizing problems, it was 0.81; Kahn, Brandt, and Whitaker, 2004), and good internal consistency for the overall measure, including the four supplemental items, was also established at 0.92 and remained consistent for the white, black and Hispanic populations (0.92, 0.93, and 0.91, respectively; Spencer et al., 2005). The BITSEA showed a 78–95 percent sensitivity and a 68–95 percent specificity when compared to the Child Behavior Checklist (CBCL) for 1.5- to 5-year-olds (Caselman and Self, 2008). The BPI was used on its own for sites that worked with children older than 3 and was combined with the BITSEA for sites that worked with children both younger than and older than 3.

To combine the two scales for use over the entire age range (1–18), we began with an exploratory factor analysis. Items were modeled as categorical using the Mplus software, and the WLSM estimator was used (Muthen and Muthen, 1998–2004). For both scales, a single-factor solution fit the data well, and items loaded strongly on the first factor. A final exploratory factor analysis (EFA) was conducted on the two scales combined, and here too the single-factor solution fit well (comparative fit index [CFI] = 0.957, nonnormed fit index [NNFI] = 0.956, root mean square error of approximation [RMSEA] = 0.047), although two items (14 and 16) from the BITSEA had very weak loadings that were just barely significant. Other than these two items, standardized loadings were large and strongly significant, ranging from 0.345 to 0.811. In the next step, we used item response theory (IRT) to create a single score for the entire age range that combined data from the two scales. The pattern of eigenvalues, predominantly strong loadings, and reasonable fit for the single-factor model provided evidence that the item set is sufficiently unidimensional for IRT calibration. Items were then calibrated using the graded response model (Samejima, 1997) in the Multilog software (Thissen, 1991). It was determined that inclusion/exclusion of the two poorly fitting items did not impact parameter estimates, so they were included in the scoring computations. Thus, a single IRT score for behavior problems was developed that calibrated the scores on these two measures across the age span. The resulting score for behavior problems is a standard score, with a mean of 0 and a standard deviation of 1. A higher score indicates more behavior problems.

Child Report of Delinquency. To assess self-reported delinquency for children ages 11–18, we selected items from and modified three instruments: the National Youth Survey (NYS), the Rochester Youth Development Study (RYDS), and the Los Angeles Family and Neighborhood Survey (LA FANS). The NYS (Elliott, 2008) was designed as a self-report instrument for youths age 11 and older, and items are used extensively by researchers to capture initiation and severity of delinquent behavior, including criminal property and violent offending. Items from the RYDS (Thornberry et al., 1998) were modified to capture delinquent behavior, primarily status offenses. The RYDS was developed for a longitudinal study of children as part of the OJJDP-funded Causes and Correlates of Delinquency Program. Finally, items from the LA FANS (Sastry and Pebley, 2003) on sexual activity initiation and frequency were included. The LA FANS is a RAND Corporation study of a representative sample of all neighborhoods and households in Los Angeles County. There were no reliability or validity data available for these measures. On this self-report instrument, children age 11 and older were asked to indicate whether they had engaged in a range of delinquent behaviors (e.g., alcohol and drug use, smoking, theft, truancy, assault). Those who marked yes for any item were asked to fill in the approximate number of times they had engaged in the behavior and the age at which they first initiated that behavior. From this information, we calculated the frequency of delinquent behaviors endorsed by children ranging from ages 0 to 18.

Social-Emotional Competence

Measures of affective strengths, school functioning, cooperation, assertion, self-control, and social and emotional competence in general were selected from four scales, two of which have different versions for different age ranges and respondents.

Caregiver Report of Child Personal-Social Competence. We used the six-item personal-social scale for children ages 0–2 from the Ages and Stages Questionnaire (ASQ; Squires, Potter, and Bricker, 1997), a development screener for children under 60 months and as young as 4 months. Items from the personal-social scale were selected from the four-month, six-month, eight-month, ten-month, 12-month, and 14-month questionnaires. The ASQ asks caregivers about the frequency (yes, sometimes, and not yet) of behaviors of their young child (e.g., Does your baby watch his/her hands? While lying on his/her back, does your baby play by grabbing his/her foot?). An age indicator was added to the instrument to aid with appropriate administration. Normative studies have found the ASQ and its subscales to be reliable. Overall Cronbach's alphas ranged from 0.56 to 0.83 for ages 4–24 months, and from 0.52 to 0.68 for the personal-social scale of the ASQ for this age group (Squires, Potter, and Bricker, 1999). The Cronbach's alphas ranged from 0.4 to 0.8, depending on age, in the present study. Prior studies showed the test to be valid, with an overall specificity of 86 percent and sensitivity of 72 percent (Squires, Potter, and Bricker, 1999). We computed a total score for this measure that can range from 0 to 60, with a higher score indicating more personal and social competence.

Caregiver Report of Child Self-Control and Child Assertion. Two scales were used to assess these domains and were combined via advanced psychometric techniques to create a measure that could be used across ages. The BITSEA (Briggs-Gowan and Carter, 2002) was used for ages 1–3 to asses social-emotional competence, with the caregiver responding to statements about the child's behavior in the past month (e.g., shows pleasure when he/she succeeds, follows rules) by rating how true or frequent each behavior is (2 = very true or often, 1 = somewhat true or sometimes, and 0 = not true or rarely). This measure has been shown to have good inter-rater reliability, test-retest reliability, and validity, with competence correlated with concurrent observed competence and predicted later competence measures (Briggs-Gowan et al., 2004). In addition, we used the Social Skills Rating System (SSRS; Gresham and Elliott,

1990) to assess cooperation (ten items), assertion (ten items), and self-control (ten items). Caregivers with preschool-age children (ages 3–5) or children in grades K–6 (ages 6–12) completed the parent-report version, which asks the caregiver to rate the frequency (2 = very often, 1 = sometimes, and 0 = never) of a series of behaviors (e.g., How often does your child use free time at home in an acceptable way? How often does your child avoid situations that are likely to result in trouble?).

The SSRS was found to be reliable in prior studies, with Cronbach's alphas of 0.90 for its social skills scale and 0.84 for problem behaviors (Gresham and Elliot, 1990). Other studies have examined convergent validity and found moderate to high correlations between the SSRS and other social competence measures, including the Woodcock-Johnson Scales of Independent Behavior (Merrell and Popinga, 1994), the Vineland Adaptive Behavior Scales (Albertus et al., 1996) and the Behavior Assessment System for Children (Flanagan et al., 1996).

In order to develop a calibrated measure that could be used across the entire age span (1–12), we began by conducting an exploratory factor analysis on these items using the Mplus software. Items were modeled as categorical, and the WLSM estimator was used (Muthen and Muthen, 1998–2004). Preliminary analyses were conducted to determine the factor structure of the instruments separately.[1] For the SSRS, results of the EFA of both the young and old versions supported the three scales used by the instrument developers (Cooperation, Assertion, and Self-Control). For the BITSEA items, there were two eigenvalues larger than 1 (4.07, 1.43), and the two-factor solution looked suitable (CFI = 0.993, NNFI = 0.989, RMSEA = 0.024), with the first factor (items 1, 10, 22, 25, 29, and 31) having content similar to the Assertion scale in the SSRS and the second factor (items 5, 13, 15, 19, and 20) having content similar to the Self-Control items in the SSRS. To confirm these findings, EFAs were conducted using data from (1) the SSRS Assertion items and factor 1 of the BITSEA items and (2) the SSRS Self-Control items and factor 2 of the BITSEA items. In both cases, analyses supported a single-factor solution. For Assertion and BITSEA factor 1, the single-factor fit was good (CFI = 0.954, NNFI = 0.947, RMSEA = 0.048), although one BITSEA item (10) did not load very strongly on the factor and did not have strong face validity. Thus, we decided to exclude this item in subsequent analyses. For Self-Control and BITSEA factor 2, the single-factor fit was also good (CFI = 0.975, NNFI = 0.971, RMSEA = 0.055), and all items loaded strongly on the single factor. Results showed that these two item sets are each sufficiently unidimensional for IRT calibration. Assertion and Self-Control items were calibrated separately using the graded IRT model (Samejima, 1997) in the Multilog software (Thissen, 1991). The resulting scores for each subscale have a mean value of 0 and a standard deviation of 1, with a higher score indicating more assertion or more self-control.

Caregiver Report of Child Cooperation. Because we were not able to combine the SSRS Cooperation Scale with the BITSEA, as described above, we kept a separate cooperation scale from the SSRS (Gresham and Elliott, 1990) for use with ages 3–12. In previous studies, the scale has been shown to be reliable, with a Cronbach's alpha of 0.81 for ages 3–5 and 0.76 for ages 6–12. In the present study, the Cronbach's alphas for caregiver reports of cooperation

[1] The two different age versions of the SSRS had to be examined separately because of the non-overlap of the ten (x2) items unique to each scale (there are 40 items in total and no data to estimate covariances between the ten unique items in each set). Similarly, the BITSEA items could only be examined together with the younger version of the SSRS. There were no common data (or reason) to examine the structure for the BITSEA and the older version of the SSRS combined.

were 0.81 (ages 3–5) and 0.86 (ages 6–12). This scale ranged from 0 to 20, with a higher score indicating more cooperation.

Child Self-Report of Assertion, Self-Control, and Cooperation. For children ages 13–18, we used the self-report version of the SSRS (Gresham and Elliott, 1990) to assess assertion, self-control, and cooperation. Questions were asked about the frequency (2 = very often, 1 = sometimes, and 0 = never) of some of the child's own behaviors (e.g., I make friends easily, I ignore classmates who are clowning around in class). Previous studies have found this scale to be reliable, with a Cronbach's alpha of 0.68 for assertion, 0.68 for self-control, and 0.67 for cooperation (Gresham and Elliott, 1990). For self-report measures administered to children ages 13–18 in this study, the Cronbach's alpha was 0.69 for assertion, 0.57 for self-control, and 0.72 for cooperation. We computed a total score for each subscale of this measure that can range from 0 to 20, with a higher score indicating more assertion, self-control, and cooperation.

Caregiver and Child Reports of Child School Functioning and Affective Strengths. We used two scales from the BERS-2 (Epstein and Sharma, 1998) to assess school functioning (nine items) and affective strengths (seven items) from the perspective of both caregivers (for children ages 6–12) and children (for children ages 11–18). For the caregiver version, we modified the instructions for use by an interviewer, and the caregiver responded to a series of statements about the child (e.g., demonstrates a sense of belonging to family, completes school tasks on time) using the provided scale (3 = very much like your child, 2 = like your child, 1 = not much like your child, and 0 = not at all like your child). Children between the ages of 11–18 were given the self-report version, responding to statements about self (e.g., my family makes me feel wanted, I do my school work on time) using the same type of scale (3 = very much like you, 2 = like you, 1 = not much like you, and 0 = not at all like you).

In a normative sample, the Cronbach's alphas for the parent report scale were 0.84 for affective strength and 0.85 for school functioning, (Epstein, 2004). The scale has also demonstrated good test-retest reliability (composite strength index of $r = 0.87$), content validity, criterion validity, and construct validity (Mooney et al., 2005). In the present study, the Cronbach's alphas for the caregiver affective strengths and school functioning were 0.76 and 0.87, respectively. In a normative sample for the youth report scale, the Cronbach's alphas were 0.80 for affective strength and 0.88 for school functioning. The scale has also demonstrated good test-retest reliability (composite strength index of $r = 0.91$), content validity, criterion validity, and construct validity (Mooney et al., 2005). In the present study, the Cronbach's alphas for internal consistency for the child self-report scales measuring affective strengths and school functioning were 0.68 and 0.76, respectively. For both versions of the scales (caregiver report and self-report), we computed a total score for each subscale that can range from 0 to 21 for the affective strength subscale and from 0 to 27 for the school functioning subscale, with a higher score indicating more affective strength and a higher level of functioning at school.

Caregiver-Child Relationship

Measures of parenting stress and family involvement were used to assess caregiver-child relationship.

Caregiver Report of Parenting Stress. To examine parenting stress, we used the Parenting Stress Index—Short Form (PSI-SF; Reitman, Currier, and Stickle, 2002). This is a 36-item measure derived from the longer Parenting Stress Index (PSI). The PSI-SF has three scales, each with 12 items: parental distress, dysfunctional parent-child interaction, and difficult child characteristics. Caregivers of children between the ages of 0 and 12 respond to statements about themselves or feelings about/interactions with their child (e.g., I often have the feeling that I cannot handle things very well, my child rarely does things for me that make me feel good) with their level of agreement with the statement (5 = strongly agree, 4 = agree, 3 = not sure, 2 = disagree, 1 = strongly disagree). In prior research, the scale was shown to have good internal consistency, with Cronbach's alphas of 0.87 for the parental distress scale, 0.80 for the parent-child dysfunctional interaction scale, 0.85 for the difficult child scale, and 0.91 for the total stress scale (Abidin, 1995). In the present study, the Cronbach's alphas were 0.87 for the parental distress scale, 0.88 for the parent-child dysfunction scale, 0.89 for the difficult child scale, and 0.94 for the total stress scale. We computed a total score for each subscale, as well as a total score, with higher scores indicating more stress for each dimension. We also identified those in our sample whose score fell in the clinical range for each dimension and for total stress.

Caregiver and Child Reports of Family Involvement. The family involvement (ten-item) scale from the BERS-2 (Epstein and Sharma, 1998) was used as a measure of caregiver-child relationship. Caregivers reported on this dimension for children ages 6–12, and children ages 11–18 completed a self-report measure. In the normative sample, the Cronbach's alpha for the caregiver report was 0.89, and for the child self-report, it was 0.80 (Epstein, 2004); in the present study, it was 0.79 and 0.77, respectively. We computed a total score for each scale ranging from 0 to 20, with a higher score indicating more family involvement.

School Readiness/Performance

Child Achievement. To assess the general domain of school readiness and performance, we used the Woodcock-Johnson III scale (WJ-III; Blackwell, 2001). We used this measure for children between the ages of 3 and 18 and chose three tests: Letter-Word Identification, Passage Comprehension, and Applied Problems. The score cards were copied into the survey, rather than being presented as separate test books. The number of items in each test ranges from 1 to 64, depending on the type of test and the child's age. Each test took approximately 3–7 minutes to complete.

The WJ-III was developed and normed with a representative 8,818 individuals from over 100 geographically diverse communities throughout the United States. The measure has been shown to have sound psychometrics, with median reliability coefficient alphas for all age groups ranging from 0.81 to 0.94, excellent reliability scores (mostly 0.90 or higher), and the individual test reliabilities mostly 0.80 or higher (McGrew and Woodcock, 2001). Growth curves of cluster scores illustrate expected developmental progressions, with steep growth from age 5 to 25 and a decline thereafter. Content, construct, and concurrent validity are supported by an extensive list of studies (McGrew and Woodcock, 2001). For each of the three tests, interviewers began with a particular item keyed to the child's age and then administered the test following instructions to establish a basal (going backward or forward until the child was correct on six items) and then to reach a ceiling (the child was incorrect on six items), following specific instructions about items and their placement on the ends of pages. If the test was not administered correctly to achieve both a basal and a ceiling, the test was not scored. Once scored, the total score was converted to an age equivalent score and then subtracted from the child's actual age to see the difference in performance on the test from what would be expected for the child's age. Positive scores indicated less readiness for school and lower school performance (age equivalent on test is lower than actual age), whereas negative scores indicate more readiness for school and higher school performance (age equivalent on test is greater than actual age).

Violence Exposure

Three measures were used to capture violence exposure in children and caregivers.

Caregiver and Child Self-Report of Juvenile Victimization. To assess exposure to violence among children ages 0–12, we used the Juvenile Victimization Questionnaire (JVQ; Hamby et al., 2004a, 2004b). The questionnaire includes several domains: conventional crime, child maltreatment, peer and sibling victimization, witnessing and indirect violence, and sexual assault. It is composed of 34 items and follow-up probes that help to assess the severity and chronicity of the event against the child (e.g., Did anyone ever hit or attack you/your child without using an object or weapon? How many times? What was the most serious injury from this?). We chose a subset of 19 items that were of the most interest[2] and modified the probes to fit the needs of the study[3] (as permitted by the developers). We also modified the wording of two items and one set of instructions to improve the clarity of the items; an additional two items were modified to include both seeing and hearing violence. The caregiver version was given to caregivers of children between the ages of 0 and 12, and the self-report version was completed by children between the ages of 11 and 18. Previous psychometric evaluation has shown good reliability and validity of both the youth and caretaker reports of the JVQ (Finkelhor et al., 2005), but no specific values were reported. We computed a total score for each subscale, as well as a total overall score, with higher scores indicating more types of violence exposure on each dimension. We did not use the information on frequency or severity of these exposures in the present study. At baseline, the survey asked about these experiences over the child's entire lifetime, and on the follow-up surveys, the survey queried about the previous six months (since the prior assessment).

Caregiver Victimization. To assess caregiver victimization, we selected and modified items from the National Victimization Crime Survey (NCVS) and the Traumatic Stress Survey. The NCVS is a national measure of crime victimization and is widely used in research. Five items from the Traumatic Stress Survey were added to include a measure for life stress related to violence. The resulting scale included two general questions (adapted from the NCVS) about whether in the past year the caregiver had been threatened or attacked by a stranger, friend, or acquaintance or by an intimate partner. If the caregiver answered yes, follow-up questions asked for additional detail on these events. A third part of the survey contains seven additional items (adapted from the Traumatic Stress Survey) that ask the respondent about her or his experience of a series of traumatic events (e.g., Did a loved one die because of an accident, homicide, or suicide?). There were no reliability or validity data available for the NCVS. We coded the resulting data for the presence or absence of domestic violence and for the presence or absence of other violence/traumatic events (non–domestic violence) to create two indicators

---

[2] We included two out of the eight items about conventional crime (assault with a weapon, assault without a weapon), all four items on child maltreatment (physical abuse by caregiver, psychological/emotional abuse, neglect, custodial interference/family abduction), one out of the six items on peer and sibling victimization (emotional bullying), three out of the seven items on sexual victimization (sexual assault by known adult, nonspecific sexual assault, sexual assault by peer), and six out of the nine items on witnessing and indirect victimization (witness to domestic violence; witness to parent assault of sibling; witness to assault with weapon; witness to assault without weapon; murder of family member or friend; exposure to random shootings, terrorism, or riots; exposure to war or ethnic conflict). We also included a question about what type of victimization occurred first and at what age.

[3] For all 17 types of victimization, we asked about the number of times it occurred. For the questions on conventional crime and physical abuse by a caregiver, we also asked what the most serious injury was (e.g., small bruise, large bruise, sprain, etc.).

of these types of experiences. At baseline, the survey asked about these experiences in the past year, and on the follow-up surveys, the survey queried about the previous six months (since the prior assessment).

Family Status Sheets

FSSs were completed at baseline, six, 12, 18, and 24 months for all families enrolled in the study. These were completed by the program if the family had received services from the Safe Start project in the previous period, even if the family was no longer participating in the research assessments. The purpose of the FSS was to document the type and amount of services received by each family in the previous period, as well as the reason that the services ended. The source of this information was staff reports based on program records. These forms were used to document Safe Start services only; families were queried about their health services more generally as part of the survey.

At baseline, the nine-item FSS captured demographic information about the child, reasons for referral to services, and date of the caregiver's and child's assessment. At six, 12, 18, and 24 months, the follow-up FSS collected information on the type and amount of Safe Start services the family received since the last assessment and whether and why services had ended (e.g., treatment/intervention satisfactorily completed; treatment/intervention goals met; family dropped out of services, lost contact, or otherwise could not continue). Caregiver status (i.e., the same or different) and placement status (i.e., whether it was the same or different and the number of placements) was also recorded at six, 12, 18, and 24 months.

The programs also recorded information on the FFS about reasons why a caregiver or child did not complete a research assessment for a particular point in time (when applicable).

Spanish-Language Translations

The assessment packets were offered in English and Spanish. Whenever possible, we used the Spanish translation available from the publisher (ASQ, BITSEA, CDI, PSI-SF, TSCC, TSCYC and WJ-III). Two measures had been translated for a different study, and we received permission from the publisher to use those Spanish translations (BERS-2 and BPI). We obtained a Spanish translation of the caregiver and child background information items from the developer of those items. For the JVQ, we received a Spanish translation of the self-report version of the measure and used that to create a Spanish translation of the caregiver report. With the SSRS, we had permission from the publisher to use the Spanish translations of the items for ages 3–5 and ages 6–12 that had been developed for another research study. We had the publisher's permission to fully translate the SSRS items for the 13- to 18-year-old assessment packet. We fully translated the child report of delinquency items and the ESI. For those measures requiring translation, we had a native Spanish speaker fully translate each measure, including the items and instructions. We then had the full translations reviewed by a second native Spanish speaker, with any differences resolved by consensus between the translator and reviewer.

Translation of the English instruments into Spanish was a considerable challenge because of anticipated variation in the Spanish-speaking populations expected to enroll in the Safe

Start programs. For example, Spanish-speaking populations in San Diego were expected to largely hail from Mexico or Central America, whereas Spanish speakers in New York City may have cultural and language ties to Puerto Rico and the Dominican Republic. It was not feasible for the research assessments to be translated into dialects of Spanish that would best suit each particular cultural and linguistic group within the study, so we instead aimed for vocabulary that could be understood by all Spanish speakers. However, since the majority of the research assessments were delivered in English and we did not conduct subgroup analyses by language or ethnicity, this issue is unlikely to affect the results.

Prioritizing Outcome Measures at Each Site

Because each site's intervention was unique, the outcome measures were prioritized differently for each site, depending on the specific targets of each intervention. Prior to analyzing the data, we examined the targets of the intervention, as described in the Safe Start process evaluation report (Schultz et al., 2010), and then we shared the prioritization with each site and asked for feedback. For instance, a site that conducted extensive case management with families would have caregiver experiences of violence and everyday problems as outcomes with higher priority, whereas a site that worked only with older children in a group format without parents would have these as lower-priority outcomes or would potentially not examine these outcomes at all. As a specific example, if the intervention primarily focused on assertion and self-control and had a secondary focus on cooperation, the site could have selected social-emotional competence as both a primary and a secondary outcome. Table 3.4 contains a summary of the prioritized outcomes by site. Because the outcomes listed cover multiple areas (e.g., social-emotional competence comprises child personal-social competence, assertion, control, and cooperation), some sites selected outcomes as both primary and secondary or tertiary, depending on the emphasis of their intervention. More information on specific measures used for primary, secondary, and tertiary outcomes for each site is presented the individual site chapters. For the sites that were delivering CPP services, feedback from different sites did not align completely, and we therefore discussed the outcomes with each site and developed a plan that was then applied to all sites.

Table 3.4
Prioritized Outcomes by Site

Site	Caregiver Resource and Personal Problems	Child PTSD Symptoms	Child Depressive Symptoms	Child Behavior/ Conduct Problems	Child Social-Emotional Competence	Caregiver-Child Relationship	Child School Readiness/ Performance	Child Violence Exposure	Caregiver Violence Exposure
Bronx	3	1	—	1	1 and 2	1	3	2	1
Broward County	3	1	1	1	2	1	3	1	1
Chelsea	3	1	2	1	2	1 and 2	2	2	3
Dallas	3	2	2	1 and 2	2	1	2	2	2
Dayton	3	1	—	1	1 and 2	1	3	1	1
Erie	3	1	2	1 and 3	1	2	1	1	2
Kalamazoo	—	1	—	1	1	2	1	3	3
Miami (IMH)	3	1	—	1	1 and 2	1	3	2	2
Miami (Heroes)	—	2	2	2 and 3	1 and 2	2	3	2	2
Multnomah County	2	2	—	2	2 and 3	1 and 2	3	1	1
Oakland	2	1	—	1	1 and 2	1	3	1	1
Providence	3	1	1	1 and 2	1 and 2	1	3	1	1
San Diego	3	1	2	1 and 2	1 and 2	2	2	1	1
San Mateo	3	1	—	1	1 and 2	1	3	2	2
Washington Heights/Inwood (CPP)	3	1	—	1	1 and 2	1	3	2	2
Washington Heights/Inwood (Kids' Club)	—	1	1	1 and 3	3	2 and 3	3	2	2

NOTES: 1 = primary outcome, 2 = secondary outcome, 3 = tertiary outcome. IMH = Infant Mental Health.

CHAPTER FOUR

Data Collection Procedures

Overview

Data sources for the outcome evaluation were primary caregiver interviews, child interviews (for ages 3 and over), and family/child-level service utilization data provided by the Safe Start program staff. All caregiver assessments were interviewer administered. Child assessments were interviewer administered for ages 3 through 10. Children ages 11 and older completed a self-administered assessment packet, but research staff was available to assist the child as needed. The sites mailed data on a monthly basis to RAND for data entry, cleaning, and analysis.

In order to standardize procedures across each of the 15 Safe Start sites, the RAND evaluation team developed detailed data collection procedures and forms. The supervisor and interviewer training manuals described each step of the data collection process. Using these manuals, the RAND team provided initial on-site data collection trainings for supervisors and research staff employed by each of the 15 Safe Start sites. The sites then implemented the data collection procedures and trained new data collection staff (when turnover occurred). The RAND team provided oversight and delivered refresher training sessions by conference call or on site, as needed.

In the remainder of this chapter, we provide a detailed description of the data collection procedures.

Data Collection Training

The 15 sites varied in their evaluation and data collection experience and prior training. In some sites, evaluation supervisors were trained and experienced researchers who were able to draw on their experience in conducting other longitudinal data collection efforts with children and families. Specifically, in five sites, data collection was managed directly by research staff within a university, research organization, or agency research office. Of the remaining ten sites, local university or research center–affiliated staff provided consultation directly to site data collection supervisors for three sites. Sites varied in the training and experience of the data collectors they employed to recruit participants and conduct research assessments. Some sites utilized existing agency staff, while others hired part-time employees or graduate students for these roles.

RAND staff delivered on-site training to data collection and supervisory staff on site. The intensity of the training was tailored somewhat, depending on the prior training and experience of the site's staff. RAND developed generic training materials applicable to all sites, worked with each site to develop its site-specific materials, and then used these materials to train data collection and supervisory staff on site. The materials included the following information:

- Generic materials:
  - overview of the study and the site's role in the national evaluation
  - general interviewing guidelines
  - general interviewing skills
  - guidelines on working with diverse populations
  - specific training with the assessment instruments and review of each instrument's specifications
  - procedures for increasing retention, including obtaining tracking and locating information for follow-ups
- Site-specific materials:
  - eligibility criteria and screening procedures
  - confidentiality agreement for data collection staff
  - IRB-approved data safeguarding plan
  - IRB-approved consent and assent procedures and forms
  - IRB-approved emergency and child abuse reporting procedures.

Data collection trainings lasted 1.5 to 2 days each. Supervisors attended the first half day that covered the procedures. The data collectors attended the full training, which included role play and practice administering the assessment instruments. The training also focused on issues of recruitment and retention strategies for data collection staff and supervisors.

Once data collection began, we fielded questions from the sites on enrollment and data collection procedures. We developed responses to these questions and periodically sent all sites a list of the frequently asked questions with detailed responses. In the case of significant data collection staff turnover, we conducted a retraining session with on-site staff.

Enrollment Procedures

As previously described in this report, each site developed its own eligibility criteria and established referral procedures with each of its referral sources. Common across all sites were the inclusion criteria of the child's exposure to violence, the availability of a guardian to provide informed consent, and the ability of the caregiver and child to understand English or Spanish. Once eligibility was confirmed, site program staff logged identifying information about the referred, or target, child. Only one child per family could participate in the study, so as to eliminate clustering of outcomes within families. While it would be possible to use multilevel modeling to account for expected within-family correlations, adding more than one child per family would have resulted in a loss of the study's power to detect intervention effects. If more than one child within the family fell within the study's eligibility criteria, each site had established its own criteria for selecting the target child who would serve as the focus of the research assessments (even if more members of the family participated in the intervention services). Many sites chose to select the child with the most recent birthday, in order to implement a roughly random selection process.

The specific procedures for obtaining consent and assent varied according to the requirements of each site's IRB. Across all sites, consent to participate in the study had to be obtained from the child's legal guardian and from the primary caregiver, if these were not the same person. A primary caregiver in each referred family was also identified to participate in the study by completing the research assessments. In some cases, this individual was not the legal guardian. Primary caregiver status was determined by asking each referred family, "Who is the person primarily responsible for this child? This is the person who makes the decisions about what's best for this child most of the time, like bedtime, when s/he goes to the doctor, what s/he eats for meals." If the legal guardian changed, the sites were instructed to secure a new signed consent form from the new legal guardian. If the primary caregiver changed, the site obtained a signed consent form from the new caregiver for his or her own participation in the study. If the child had not lived with the caregiver completing the assessment for 30 days, the sites were asked to delay conducting the assessment and enrolling the child until the child and caregiver had lived together for 30 days.

Assent from children was only sought after the consent from adults was obtained. Children ages 3–17 were asked to complete an assent process to participate in the study. In most cases, young children (ages 3–6) provided verbal assent (which was documented in writing by the data collector), and older children assented in writing. Sites determined the method of assent (i.e., verbal or written) based on local IRB requirements and state laws. RAND's IRB required that the assent protocol inform children that they could decline participation in the study, even if their parent/guardian consented.

All sites offered incentives to the caregivers for study participation. In most cases, details on incentives were outlined in the consent protocol. Sites varied on the type and amount of incentives offered to participants. Nine of the 15 sites provided gift cards, and the other six made cash payments to the participants. Incentive amounts ranged from $20 to $60 for each completed caregiver assessment. Three sites increased the payment amount by $5 for each successively completed caregiver assessment. Two sites offered a bonus incentive if all follow-up assessments were completed.

Those consenting to participate were then enrolled in the study. Sites' enrollment procedures varied based on their research design. For sites using a comparison group design, research group assignment was determined by the setting or source of the referral. Thus, participating families and staff knew their actual group assignment prior to consenting to the study and completing the baseline assessments.

Sites using a randomized design did not determine group assignment until after the baseline assessment with the caregiver (and child, when applicable) was complete. Sites then followed a standardized protocol for group assignment that sought to equalize the groups on child age using a block randomized design. The randomization design stratified age into a maximum of four possible groups, with the number of groups dependent on the age range of the site:

1. 0–2
2. 3–6
3. 7–12
4. 13–18.

For each site, RAND generated a separate random list of group assignments within each age block. For example, one site's random group assignment list for the first six children ages

3–6 may have been control, control, treatment, control, treatment, treatment. RAND then assigned a unique sequential study identification number to each of these conditions. Sites were provided with a set of color-coded envelopes that corresponded to each age strata applicable to its study. Each envelope was labeled on the outside with the RAND-assigned unique study identification number. After the baseline assessment was completed, site research staff would select the next number in the appropriate age strata sequence and open the corresponding envelope. Its contents would reveal the family's assignment to the treatment or control group, and the family would be assigned the number on the envelope as their unique identifier.

RAND monitored the randomization process closely to ensure that identification numbers were being assigned sequentially within age group and that group assignment was proceeding according to design. Any deviations from the random assignment process (e.g., withdrawal after randomization) are noted in the outcomes report for each site.

Completing and Processing Assessments

As discussed in Chapter Two, the specific contents of the caregiver and child assessments varied by the age of the target child. Interviewers were trained to select the age-appropriate assessment packet to administer at baseline and to administer the same assessment packet again at six months, even if the child had "aged in" to the next assessment. For the 12-, 18-, and 24-month assessment points, assessment packet selection was based solely on the child's age at the time of the assessment. Assessments were usually administered in person, though infrequently some assessments needed to be completed by phone. All caregiver assessments and assessments for children ages 3 through 10 were interviewer administered. Children age 11 and older were given self-administered assessments, with the exception of the subtests of the Woodcock-Johnson instrument (which was always interviewer administered). When administering child assessments, the guidelines was that the parent or caregiver not be in the room during verbally administered portions, so long as the child was comfortable with his or her absence. For older children, a parent or caregiver could be present for self-administered portions, provided that he or she did not sit or stand where the child's answers were visible.

For the baseline assessments, every instrument in the caregiver assessment needed to be completed for the family to be fully enrolled in the study and to remain in the study. If a child assessment could not be completed in whole or in part at the baseline, sites were instructed to consult with us to determine whether the family could remain in the study. In the majority of circumstances, we allowed the family to remain in the study. If the two assessments (caregiver and child) were separated in time, we allowed up to 30 days to complete the second assessment. For the follow-up assessments, if the caregiver and/or child began the assessment but could not complete all or part, families remained in the study and were tracked in an attempt to complete the next time point's follow-up assessment.

All assessments were administered in Spanish or English, with interviewers selecting the appropriate primary language based on which the respondent preferred or spoke most frequently. For each English and Spanish assessment, RAND developed a detailed set of specifications that provided item-level instructions to interviewers. These included whether interviewers could offer other words if a respondent asked for question clarification and, if so, what other words or clarification should be offered, as well as how to code specific responses. As needed, interviewers also coded item refusals, indicating the reason the item was refused.

At each follow-up assessment point, site research or program staff completed an FSS based on program records about the type and amount of services received by the family, as well as reasons for missed assessments, if applicable. The sites were asked to complete a follow-up FSS at each subsequent time point for every family who was enrolled in the study, regardless of whether the assessment was completed.

On a monthly basis, each site would bundle together completed assessments and FSSs and submit them via mail to RAND. All data were coded by identification number only, and only sites possessed the ability to uniquely identify study participants. Each shipment of data from the sites was inventoried on arrival against a list of packets and identification numbers emailed by the site at the time of the shipment. RAND research staff reviewed each submitted assessment packet and worked with sites to address any missing data or clarify any inconsistent responses. When a pattern of errors was detected, RAND staff would arrange refresher trainings or other responses to assist a site in reducing its data collection errors. All packet data were scanned electronically into a database on a rolling basis.

RAND research staff also constructed a tracking database to log each baseline and follow-up assessments as it was received. This database was used to generate monthly reports for each site about which study identification numbers were coming due for a follow-up assessment and which assessment packet should be used, based on the age of the child. This database was also used to confirm that the appropriate assessment packet was used at each time point.

Data Cleaning

The guidelines set out for data collection were not always achieved, resulting in data cleaning that was conducted at RAND on a routine and ongoing basis. The main issues related to data cleaning, and how issues were resolved, are listed below:

- Questions about birthdates, assessment dates and wave, and intervention group were resolved on delivery to RAND by working with the site to answer questions and clean data prior to scanning. Missing pages of assessment packets were handled in the same way. Responses for primary language spoken at home and race/ethnicity were changed to more accurately reflect information respondents provided in the "other" category. For example, in one case a respondent did not check "Hispanic" for race/ethnicity and instead checked "other," writing in "El Salvadoran." This response was changed to "Hispanic" from "other." The Woodcock-Johnson tests were examined on delivery to RAND to determine if they could be scored. Those that could not be scored were noted in an error database to ensure that scores generated in the programming process would be set to "missing." In addition, programming code was set to catch additional tests that did not include either the basal or ceiling, and those were set to "missing" as well.
- In some cases, the assessment delivered to the child and/or caregiver was not the appropriate one for the child's age. In these cases, the specific assessments that were collected in error were set to "missing" in the database and thus are excluded from analysis.
- Data collection procedures stipulated that caregiver and child assessments be completed within 30 days of each other. However, in some cases the lag time between the two assessments was longer (see Table 4.1). In the final sample, we included caregiver and child assessments that were completed within 90 days of each other in order to standardize the

observation window for all assessments. Three cases that were outside of the 90-day lag time; for these, only the child assessment was excluded in the analysis and dropped from the public use dataset, since the child assessment contained less data than the caregiver assessment.

- Data collection procedures stipulated that assessments be collected within a window of two weeks prior to and eight weeks after the target date (of six, 12, 18, or 24 months after the baseline assessment). However, in some cases the assessment was completed outside of this window (see Table 4.2). In the final sample, we included assessments that were completed within an expanded window of 2.5 months prior to and four months after the target date to maximize the amount of data available for analyses.

Implementation of Study Procedures

Overall, the data collection procedures were successfully implemented, but there were some key challenges. One challenge was balancing the length of the assessment with the burden placed on respondents. There were concerns that the length of assessments may be too much for families with young children to successfully complete and that this would pose a barrier to their participation. As data collection progressed, it appeared that the assessment length was not a barrier to participation. Another issue related to the content of the assessments was concern about asking directly about violence exposure and direct victimization of children in the research assessments. In practice, the presence of these items did not appear to negatively influence participation in the study or individual assessments. Data collection protocols had to be carefully developed (based on IRB-approved procedures and guidelines) in the event that violence toward a child was detected during the research assessment. Training and monitoring procedures for the implementation of these guidelines were put into place, but ultimately very few incidents were detected that required IRB-related involvement.

Data quality was a minor issue. We observed data collection errors in over 2,000 surveys (about 18 percent of the total number of surveys). Some of the errors related to data entry (e.g., incorrect data, discrepancy in data, missing data), survey administration (e.g., incorrect administration of survey items, incorrect survey packet or form used), and survey processing (e.g., submission of multiple versions of surveys, missing all or part of survey forms).

The most challenging instrument for administration was the Woodcock-Johnson instrument measuring school readiness or performance. Many of the survey administration errors referenced above involved the Woodcock-Johnson instrument. Specifically, sites administered too many or too few items in sequence, or items were skipped. The specifics of administration are complicated (relative to the rest of the assessment), involving the interviewer presenting the child with specific materials to look at or read and beginning or ending with different ques-

Table 4.1
Lag Between Caregiver and Child Assessments

	0–30 Days	31–45 Days	46–60 Days	61–75 Days	76–90 Days	> 90 Days
Number	745	81	34	14	6	3*

* For these cases, we excluded the child assessment from the outcomes analysis.

Table 4.2
Time Outside of the Original Data Collection Window

	1–14 Days	15–30 Days	31–45 Days	46–60 Days	> 60 Days
Number of caregiver assessments	401	119	40	19	14*
Number of child assessments	160	45	21	10	7*

* We excluded these cases from the outcomes analysis.

tions depending on the child's age and ability. The RAND research team continually monitored the submitted assessment packets and discovered that data collection staff at a number of sites required retraining and closer supervision on the administration of the Woodcock-Johnson instrument. The errors appeared to be random administrator error, rather than related to a child's performance on the tests. However, the high number of errors in the administration of the Woodcock-Johnson instrument reduced the number of valid tests collected.

Generally, the data collection went quite well for a field study utilizing data collection staff with varying levels of prior experience and training on collecting data or conducting assessments. There were occasional problems, such as a sibling being assessed at a follow-up time period, rather than the original target child, because of communication issues between the core program staff and the assessors. In a small number of other cases, families were enrolled that were later determined to be ineligible. In both situations, the data were removed from the study.

In the early months of study enrollment, there was some revision in the method used to select the target child for the evaluation component (when there were multiple age-eligible children in the family). Most sites had initially been trained to select the child with the most recent birthday to make the selection a semi-random process. Over time, some sites revised their protocols to use some more intentional criterion for this selection—e.g., the child that the caregiver selects as the most in need of services. Data collection staff were then retrained on selection of the appropriate target child.

In all controlled trials, randomization can be a challenge, but the Safe Start sites were able to execute the randomization procedures with a great degree of success. With one exception, the randomization procedures were well adhered to by the sites for the entire study period, or, after some initial problems were identified, the procedures were corrected. In the site that did not adhere to the randomization, the exact reasons are unclear, though it appears that clinical staff ignored the randomization and served families with all available interventions.

Oversight via the IRB for this study was complex, and it broke new ground in establishing coordination across the different IRBs and procedures for monitoring of the study. Sites had varying levels of familiarity with such issues as data collection, confidentiality of research data, the distinction between study data and clinical records, quality monitoring for service delivery and study procedures, and the like.

As will be discussed in Chapter Six, the funding for the national evaluation ended prematurely because of a lack of a Congressional reappropriation. As a result, data collection had to end before the 24-month study window had passed for some enrolled families. Consequently, follow-up had to be cut short before one or more follow-up assessments could be completed, although four sites were able to extend data collection beyond the funded period. Sites worked with the RAND research team to develop a plan for notifying families of the end of the data collection. The plans were submitted to and approved by both RAND's IRB and each site's local IRB before execution.

CHAPTER FIVE

General Analytic Approach

Each of the 15 sites developed its own research design or designs as part of the Green Light process. In this section, we discuss the general designs at the sites, power analyses, and analytic strategies for the different types of designs and for handling issues related to missing data, multiple tests of significance, and low numbers of participants in cells. This chapter gives a general overview of these strategies, with site-specific details appearing in each of the respective site reports.

Overview of Site Research Designs

Table 5.1 presents the evaluation designs employed at each site. As can be seen in the table, the majority of sites utilized randomized controlled designs, the most definitive type of design in examining outcomes resulting from an intervention.

General Strategy for Randomized Control Group Experiments

The majority of sites planned a randomized controlled trial to examine intervention effects. As part of the Green Light process, we worked with sites to ensure that participants would be selected in an unbiased fashion and fully assessed prior to randomization. We developed the randomization procedures, as described in Chapter Four, so that sites could perform this task without bias and with a similar distribution of ages in each group.

One site (Kalamazoo, Michigan) utilized a clustered randomized design in which classrooms rather than individuals were assigned to the intervention or control condition. We worked with this site to randomize or assign classrooms within location and then adjusted for clustering within the analysis.

Three sites (Washington Heights/Inwood, part of Miami's IMH evaluation that included court-referred families, and Broward County) planned a wait-list design for the control group, in which the control group was to be offered intervention services after the six-month follow-up assessment. In these cases, examination of the six-month outcome data was the primary interest and is highlighted in the report. However, the Washington Heights/Inwood design was not implemented as planned, making it difficult to draw inferences from the data (see the Washington Heights/Inwood site report for a detailed description).

General Strategy for Quasi-Experimental Comparison Group Designs

Several sites planned a quasi-experimental design with a comparison group drawn from a clinic, shelter, or agency in the same or similar community. As part of the Green Light process

Table 5.1
Sites' Planned Research Designs

Site	Randomized Study	Quasi-Experimental Study
Bronx	X	
Broward County	X (wait list)	
Chelsea		X
Dallas	X	
Dayton	X	
Erie	X	
Kalamazoo	X (cluster-randomized)	
Miami (IMH)	X	X
Miami (Heroes)		X
Multnomah County		X
Oakland	X	
Providence Tier 2		X
Providence Tier 3	X	
San Diego	X	
San Mateo	X	
Washington Heights/ Inwood (CPP)	X (wait list)	
Washington Heights/ Inwood (Kids' Club)	X (wait list)	

and process evaluation (Schultz et al., 2010), we described the extent to which the comparison groups seemed similar to, or different from, the intervention groups. When more than one comparison site was used, we planned to control for clustering within sites.

Sites with Two or More Interventions

Three sites delivered more than one intervention to different types of families (Providence) or to different age groups (Miami and Washington Heights/Inwood). In each case, the different interventions were treated as separate studies occurring within the same site, since no overlap in families receiving services was planned.

Power Analyses

By definition, statistical power is the ability to detect an intervention effect, if one exists. Thus, higher levels of statistical power allow us to draw firmer conclusions about the effectiveness of the site's interventions. With inadequate statistical power, the results of statistical tests become hard to interpret. For example, lack of a statistically significant intervention effect could either mean that the program was not effective or that an effect was present but the statistical test was unable to detect it because of the lack of power.

Generally, three things contribute to statistical power: research design, the size of the program's effect, and the sample size. Regarding research design, random assignment to treatment and control groups yields the most power, compared with a design with treatment and comparison groups that are not or are only partially randomized. Regarding the size of the program's effect, the larger the effect, the easier it is to detect. This means that it is easier to find a statistically significant effect (i.e., to have more power) for interventions that create a very large change on the outcomes measured, compared with interventions that create a small change on the outcomes. For example, observing a large effect in this evaluation is more likely for interventions that directly work with children around the key outcomes measured in the assessment packet and less likely for those interventions that are more indirect (e.g., those that work mostly with parents or caregivers to improve child outcomes). Regarding sample size, the power calculation depends on how many families are in the two groups. The more families a study has, the more power the study has to detect as statistically significant a given effect size. Very large numbers of families make power a nonissue.

Effect Size and Sample Size

Effect size refers to how much of an impact the intervention has on an outcome among participants in the intervention group and is commonly used as a way to describe the power of a study. The effect size is a standardized measure of the strength of association between an intervention and an outcome and is defined as the average difference in an outcome between the intervention and control groups divided by the common standard error. The effect size measure is commonly classified as small if it is about 0.2, medium if it is about 0.5, and large if it is about 0.8 (Cohen, 1988). If an intervention has a big effect on participants (or, more accurately, the outcomes being measured in the study), this is more easily observed with smaller numbers of families in a study. Small intervention effects require more participants to be detectable with statistical tests. The convention in the field is to strive for enough statistical power such that the statistical test has at least an 80-percent chance of detecting the effect size that a researcher might expect to observe. Typically, researchers use the existing literature to gauge how large an effect might be anticipated for a given intervention. In the Safe Start context, however, the size of the effect anticipated for the different site interventions was difficult to gauge because of the lack of existing research on these kinds of programs. Nonetheless, for each site, we gleaned what we could from the available literature to estimate what minimum effect size could potentially be observed in the evaluation (Table 5.2).

Power Analysis Summary

Table 5.2 shows the research design, expected intervention effect size, and sample size required to achieve 80-percent power to detect the expected intervention effect size for each site. In Chapter Six of this report, we will present the results of the enrollment and retention in each site, in comparison with the numbers needed to achieve power based on this analysis. This table highlights the relationship between effect sizes and sample size for a given study type.

Table 5.2
Site Research Designs, Estimated Effect Sizes, and Proposed Sample Sizes

Site	Research Design	Estimated Effect Size	Required Sample Size for 80% Power
Bronx	RCT	Medium	200
Broward County	RCT (wait list)	Medium	200
Chelsea	Comparison	Medium	270
Dallas	RCT	Large	60
Dayton	RCT	Medium	200
Erie	RCT	Medium	200
Kalamazoo	Cluster randomized trial	Small	510[a]
Miami (IMH)	Mixed	Medium	270
Miami (Heroes)	Comparison	Medium	270
Multnomah County	Comparison	Small	680
Oakland	RCT	Medium	200
Providence Tier 2	Comparison	Small	680
Providence Tier 3	RCT	Medium	200
San Diego	RCT	Small	510
San Mateo	RCT	Medium	200
Washington Heights/ Inwood (CPP)	RCT (wait list)	Medium	200
Washington Heights/ Inwood (Kids' Club)	RCT (wait list)	Medium	200

[a] Kalamazoo's clustered design would require even more participants, but since we did not have a good estimate of the intra-class correlation, we present the unclustered power analysis in this chapter.

NOTE: RCT = randomized controlled trial.

Namely, as the expected intervention effect size increases, the required sample size for a given type of study design decreases.

During implementation, sites had difficulty meeting their enrollment and retention goals, as will be discussed in more detail in Chapter Six and in each site report. Moreover, the evaluation ended early because of funding constraints when the appropriation for Safe Start was curtailed and the national evaluation was not fully funded. Because of issues with under-recruitment, attrition, and the premature end of the evaluation, in most sites the retained sample was smaller than the sample needed for the power to detect the minimum observable effect. That is, most of the studies were underpowered for the evaluation. We therefore explain in each site report the chances of detecting the intervention effect given the sample in the study as a way of interpreting the findings within each evaluation.

Issues with statistical power were further compounded by two additional factors. First, since children differed in age within the different studies, and some sites served a broad age range, the data available on some measures were scant because there were few children in the age range eligible to complete that measure. For instance, a site could have a certain amount of power to detect differences for measures used for the full sample but lower power for measures that were completed by a subsample in a particular age range. Second, multiple statistical tests were used in this study to evaluate outcomes, and thus corrections for multiple testing were required. This further reduced power across all site evaluations.

Analysis Plan

The analysis plan for each site was similar but was constrained at each site by the available sample size. Sample size depended not only on enrollment and retention but also on the number of children at a particular age (and therefore given a particular measure at the assessment point), as well as on the quality of the data and results of data cleaning. Thus, the analysis for a particular measure could differ from other measures within a site.

The general analysis plan begins with descriptions of the sample and services delivered within the project. This includes a description of the numbers of families enrolled and retained in a group over time, a description of the child and caregiver characteristics and outcomes at baseline that compares those in the intervention and comparison/control groups, and a description of the services received by those families in the intervention group. We follow this by examination of the outcomes of interest over time. We compare means within groups across time using t-tests, compare groups via chi-square or t-tests at each time point, and examine differences in differences to compare the two groups on mean changes over time between baseline and follow-up assessments (when the sample size is at least ten per group). When feasible with the sample size (when the sample size is at least 20 per group), we conduct regressions to examine these differences in differences while controlling for demographics and baseline violence exposure.

Descriptive analyses at baseline were conducted to summarize the sample characteristics: age, gender, race/ethnicity, caregiver-child relationship, the family income level, and the child's violence exposure at baseline, as well as for all of the outcomes measured in the study. We compare the intervention and control groups via t-tests or chi-squares (depending on the type of variable of interest, continuous or categorical) to ensure that the two groups were roughly comparable, as that was the goal of the randomization performed. In this section, we also investigate the baseline status of families on two outcome variables to describe the severity of symptoms on average by children and parents prior to the intervention. We also examined differences between the intervention and control/comparison group at baseline for the primary, secondary, and tertiary outcomes.

Dosage or uptake of care was described for each site in terms of the percentage of study families in services; the average, median, and range of services (sessions, hours, or days); and the distribution of services. The dosage information was compiled for all families with service information at the six-month assessment point, regardless of whether they had a completed six-month assessment. For this sample, the dosage table compiles all services received throughout the study follow-up. We also described dosage for each site's analytic sample, summing only those services received during that period. For sites with a large enough analytic sample, we compiled a summary dosage score and, based on the distribution, created a variable to indicate whether families who received services received an overall low, medium, or high dosage of the services as a succinct way to characterize the level of services received. This variable was used in exploring the impact of services on families as described in the "Impact of Different Dosages of the Intervention on Those Who Received Treatment" section.

Differences between groups at each follow-up were described next, with follow-up estimates of primary, secondary, and tertiary outcomes for both groups (when the sample size is greater than or equal to five per cell) and simple t-test or chi-square test contrasts between intervention group and control group (when the sample size in each group is greater or equal to ten, for a total of 20 or more). Because of the small sample sizes, we conducted sensitivity analyses using nonparametric tests (Fisher's exact test and the McNemar test for categorical outcomes and the Wilcoxon rank test for continuous outcomes) to test the contrasts. In sites that had differential attrition between the intervention and control/comparison groups, we examined differences between those that were lost to follow-up and those that were retained in terms of their demographic characteristics, as well as their scores on outcomes measures at baseline, using t-tests and chi-square statistics.

Differences within groups over time are described next, with paired t-tests comparing individuals at each follow-up wave to his or her own score at the baseline assessment (when the sample size in each group is greater or equal to ten, for a total of 20 or more).

Intervention effects over time were examined when possible, depending on the size of the groups, using an intent-to-treat approach in which all families allocated to the intervention were compared to all those allocated to the control group, regardless of the actual amount of intervention received in the intervention group.

In sites with at least 20 per group at one of the follow-up points, we present differences between children in the intervention and control classrooms at six, 12, 18, and 24 months. Because any change in outcomes observed can potentially be the result of a time trend observed in all children in the study, a difference-in-difference method was used to assess the unadjusted impact of the program (when the sample size was greater than or equal to 20 in each group). With continuous outcomes, the unadjusted difference in difference is the difference between the average change in a child's outcome from baseline to follow-up between the treatment and the control groups. For dichotomous outcomes (e.g., caregiver report of any domestic violence—yes or no), the unadjusted difference-in-difference is the difference between the proportion of yes outcomes from baseline to follow-up, contrasted between the treatment and the control group.

When analyzing continuous outcomes, we also conducted multiple linear regressions on the outcomes to test for the adjusted difference in difference via main effects and the interaction between intervention status and time after controlling for baseline characteristics (child age, gender, race, and exposure to violence), assuming that the sample size was at least 20 per group. For the dichotomous outcomes, a linear probability regression model was conducted with the same main effects and interactions, with the adjusted difference in difference estimating the difference in probability in the dichotomous outcome. The baseline characteristics were selected to correct for any potential imbalance in the groups by relevant demographic characteristics.

Impact of different dosages of the intervention on those who received treatment were also examined. First, we conducted descriptive statistics to examine changes over time for those in the intervention group that received low, medium, or high dosages of the intervention services. Since groups receiving different level of services differed in terms of their baseline level of severity, a cause for concern of a possible compliance imbalance, we created matched control groups for each that closely approximated the group receiving the given service dosage, based on the baseline severity of the variable being examined. The method of propensity score was used to estimate, for example, the likelihood of a participant receiving a low dosage versus being in the control group, and every low-dosage participant was matched to control participants with similar propensity. Participants with no good match in the control group were dropped from the dosage match analysis. We then compared each dosage group to its matched control group using a difference in difference technique with a t- or chi-square test when the sample size was greater than or equal to ten in each group. As these groups were matched based on baseline level of severity, no additional adjustment was essential for inference. Second, in a sensitivity analysis, we also explored the impact of dosage by using the continuous variable of total dosage in multiple linear regressions as described earlier (when the sample size allowed it), adding the dosage variable along with the other control variables to predict primary outcomes. Since the effects of these sensitivity analyses did not differ substantially from the analyses described above, we chose not to present data from this later method.

Summary of Analytic Strategies Possible with Differing Samples

To summarize, our ability to analyze the data depended largely on the size of the samples available for each measure, at each time point, and for each group (intervention or control/comparison). For sites with more data, we were able to draw stronger inferences (even if not significant) about intervention effects than for sites with less data. In some cases, our ability to analyze the data differed measure by measure, and, thus, some measures remained untested, whereas others were tested more rigorously. Table 5.3 summarizes the analytic methods we employed and the types of inferences that could be drawn for each, according to the sample size available.

Table 5.3
Analysis and Inferences According to Sample Size

Sample Size	Analytic Methods	Inferences That Could Be Drawn If There Is Adequate Power to Detect Effects
At least five per cell	Means/no comparison	Estimates of group means for descriptive purposes only
At least ten per group	T-test or chi-square comparing groups	Compare groups at a time point
	Paired t-test over time, within groups	Determine if there are any differences within groups, over time
	Differences in differences or proportions	Determine if changes over time are different between groups and if changes can be attributed to the intervention (assuming that the groups are comparable)
At least 20 per group	Multiple linear regressions, adjusting for demographics	Determine if there is an intervention effect, controlling for background characteristics
	Dosage analysis using propensity score matching	Determine if changes over time are different between groups at varying dosages of intervention after controlling for dosage selection bias that can lead to only severe cases receiving more service

Guidelines Used Across Sites

To ensure that the analyses were as similar as possible across sites but that we did not present any analyses that would be inappropriate for a site, we developed a few guidelines that are used across all the site reports. They are as follows:

- Descriptive statistics related to outcome variables are not presented when the cell size is less than five, in order to preserve the privacy of responses of families that participated in the study.
- Contrasts between groups (t-tests and chi-squares) are not presented when either group has less than ten observations, as the contrasts would be likely to be unreliable at this size.
- Modeling of outcomes in regressions are not presented when either group has less than 20 observations, as many child characteristics are controlled for and the results are likely to be unreliable with wide confidence intervals.

Missing Data

When dealing with child outcomes based on multiple item responses, we followed the missing-items scoring rules for specific scales, which in many cases provided ways to score the assessment if a small number of missing items were present. For instance, a scale consisting of 20 items might allow scoring if 17 or more items were present, by deriving the average item response and multiplying by 20. In cases where all items were missing, the outcome assessment score was set to missing and the case was dropped in the analysis of that outcome, as these cases are infrequent in the data.

Avoiding False Discovery with Multiple Comparisons

When conducting large numbers of simultaneous hypothesis tests, as we did in this study, it is important to account for the possibility that some results will achieve statistical significance simply by chance. The use of a traditional 95-percent confidence interval, for example, will result in one out of 20 comparisons achieving statistical significance as a result of random error or chance. Adjustments should therefore be made to account for false positives when large numbers of comparisons are made. As noted earlier, the need to make corrections for multiple tests further constrains the power of these studies to detect intervention effects.

This report addresses false positives using the False Discovery Rate (FDR) method (Benjamini and Hochberg, 1995), which allows the analyst to bound the expected fraction of rejected null hypotheses that are mistakenly rejected (i.e., that are "false discoveries"). The rejection decision for each hypothesis in the family of tests is a simple function of the rank of the p-value of the test, the total number of tests, and the chosen false discovery rate.

As described in Chapter Three of this report, we determined the primary, secondary, and tertiary outcomes for each intervention a priori and vetted the prioritization of outcome with sites. Our assessments of statistical significance were based on applying the FDR procedure separately to all of the primary, secondary, and tertiary outcome tests in this report using a false discovery rate of 0.05. Thus, the cut-scores used to determine significance differ for each set of analyses, depending on the number of tests conducted. In each site report, we give information about the p-values required to determine significance. However, we also present information about nonsignificant trends observed between $p < 0.05$ and the FDR cutoff in order to indicate those results that are approaching statistical significance.

CHAPTER SIX

Overview of Outcome Evaluation Across Sites

In this chapter, we review the outcome data collected across the 14 sites that participated fully in the national evaluation, discussing characteristics of enrollees, as well as patterns of enrollment, retention, power, and outcomes that were observed.

Characteristics of Enrollees Across Sites

As noted earlier in this report, there was a good deal of variation across the SSPA sites, including their target populations for programs. Although all of the programs sought to improve outcomes for children exposed to violence, their use of different settings, focus on different age ranges and types of violence, and varying referral streams resulted in great diversity in the families who enrolled in Safe Start.

Table 6.1 displays some characteristics of families included in the evaluation at each site. Note that sites also served families outside of the evaluation, but this report focuses on those enrolled in the evaluation only. For reasons including difficulty recruiting families into and retaining families in the Safe Start evaluations (discussed more thoroughly in each site report), as well as different time lines for the different sites, the number of families enrolled at each site ranged from a low of 19 families to a high of 436 families. Each family identified one child to be enrolled in the evaluation (i.e., the target child). Both boys and girls were identified as the target child for purposes of the evaluation, but there was some variability in sites' gender distribution, with 35–63 percent of child participants being male across the sites. The average age of the target child across the sites varied from 1.7 years to 8.7 years, largely because of each program's design and eligibility criteria. While the race and ethnicity varied a good deal across sites, the majority of sites enrolled primarily racial/ethnic minority (black, Hispanic, and other nonwhite) families.[1] Sites also consistently enrolled impoverished families, although comparisons are difficult because of differences in the cost of living across the sites.

Children in families enrolled in the studies also varied a good deal in terms of their exposure to violence at the baseline assessment. Enrolled children were reported to have been exposed to an average of between 1.9 and 5.0 different types of violent events in their lifetime at the beginning of the study. Some of the variability is undoubtedly due to the age of the children enrolled, with younger children having less time to be exposed to violence, but site differences were also apparent. An even larger difference across sites is seen in the percent of children enrolled whose parents reported PTSD symptoms in the range that is considered significant.

[1] Erie, Pa., was the only site that primarily served white families.

Table 6.1
Baseline Characteristics of Enrolled Families by Site

Safe Start Program	Number of Families Enrolled in Evaluation	Gender of Target Child (% male)	Age of Child	Average Violence Exposure of Target Child (number of types of events)	Race/Ethnicity of Caregiver			Family Income Level	Percentage of Children in the Significant Range for CR of PTSD Symptoms	Percentage of Caregivers in the Clinical Range for Total Parenting Stress
					% Hispanic	% Black	% Other (nonwhite)	% ≤$15,000 in Annual Household Income		
Bronx	166	63%	4.3	3.5	69%	16%	15%	77%	49%	73%
Broward County	201	44%	3.9	2.1	6%	40%	40%	40%	28%	35%
Chelsea	82	60%	8.1	3.0	55%	4%	26%	62%	38%	81%
Dallas	85	48%	5.4	5.0	13%	54%	24%	73%	48%	71%
Dayton	55	53%	1.7	2.7	4%	49%	22%	78%	43%	40%
Erie	166	42%	6.3	4.9	1%	13%	21%	39%	55%	53%
Kalamazoo	436	48%	3.9	2.8	10%	46%	23%	59%	8%	29%
Miami (Heroes)	52	50%	7.9	3.7	4%	52%	39%	89%	25%	46%
Miami (IMH)	90	57%	2.1	1.9	3%	57%	38%	86%	8%	21%
Multnomah County	43	35%	3.6	2.9	40%	7%	23%	43%	23%	30%
Oakland	85	44%	3.4	2.6	54%	18%	24%	68%	27%	53%
Providence (Tier 2)	19	47%	4.4	3.8	0%	5%	68%	89%	33%	68%
Providence (Tier 3)	58	47%	8.0	4.8	43%	14%	26%	61%	41%	61%
San Diego	104	43%	6.5	2.4	57%	9%	27%	59%	21%	40%
San Mateo	69	45%	4.7	3.7	45%	16%	30%	15%	40%	57%
Washington Heights/ Inwood (CPP)	38	55%	4.1	3.0	74%	13%	13%	82%	45%	74%
Washington Heights/ Inwood (Kids' Club)	31	42%	8.7	3.3	84%	3%	6%	64%	24%	61%
All Sites	1,741	48%	4.7	3.2	25%	30%	26%	59%	28%	46%

NOTE: CR = Caregiver Report.

Sites varied from 8 to 55 percent on this measure. Caregivers' reports of their own parenting stress also varied considerably, with a range of 21 to 81 percent reporting stress that falls in the clinical range at baseline. These latter two factors are important to note in interpreting the results of the outcomes evaluations at each site, because families who enter programs reporting low levels of stress and few child symptoms have less room to change as a result of the evaluation, making the observation of improvements difficult.

Summary of Enrollment Across Sites

During implementation, sites had difficulty meeting their enrollment goals. In addition, data collection time lines were variable because of different start-up periods and adjustments to the time line and scope of data collection for some sites. For instance, Multnomah County discontinued enrollment in its study about two months before the other sites and stopped data collection entirely about eight months before the other sites. Each site time line is detailed in the results appendixes.

Nearly all of the sites enrolled far fewer participants than planned, and most enrolled fewer than would be needed for a well-powered study, as explained in Chapter Five. However, many of them met or exceeded typical service retention rates for mental health programs. Research estimates that 40 to 60 percent of children receiving outpatient mental health services attend few sessions and drop out quickly (Gopalan et al., 2010). A report of over 100 studies of psychotherapy attrition found an average treatment dropout rate of nearly 50 percent (Wierzbicki and Pekarik, 1993). In addition, retention rates for services delivered in urban areas, like the communities in which many of the SSPA programs operated, are as low as 9 percent after a three-month period (McKay and Bannon, 2004).

Figure 6.1 shows the actual enrollment by group for the sites with randomized control designs, comparing the actual enrollment with the target enrollment needed for power, assuming an 80-percent retention rate. For the two sites where we expected small intervention effect sizes, only Kalamazoo came close to enrolling the 319 families per group (at least 638 total) required in the study to have an 80-percent power to detect a small intervention effect. Kalamazoo enrolled a total of 436 families and likely needed even more than the number projected in Table 5.2 because of its cluster randomized design. San Diego enrolled only about 16 percent of the sample size required to detect a small intervention effect. For sites where we expected a medium intervention effect, Broward was the only site that enrolled close to the 250 families necessary to have an 80-percent chance of detecting a medium intervention effect (assuming an 80-percent retention rate). Erie and the Bronx both enrolled a total of 166 families, which was 66 percent of the sample size needed to detect a medium intervention effect, given an 80-percent retention rate. The remaining sites where we expected a medium intervention effect size enrolled from 22 to 34 percent of what was needed to detect a medium intervention effect. Dallas was the only site where a large intervention effect was expected. Dallas enrolled a total of 85 families, which was more than the sample size of 75 families required to have an 80-percent chance of detecting a large intervention effect (assuming an 80-percent retention rate). Some of the reasons for the enrollment challenges experienced by the sites with randomized control designs are described later in this section.

Several sites employed quasi-experimental comparison group designs. Figure 6.2 shows the actual enrollment by group for the sites with quasi-experimental designs. For the Chelsea

Figure 6.1
Required Versus Actual Enrollment for Sites with Randomized Control Trials

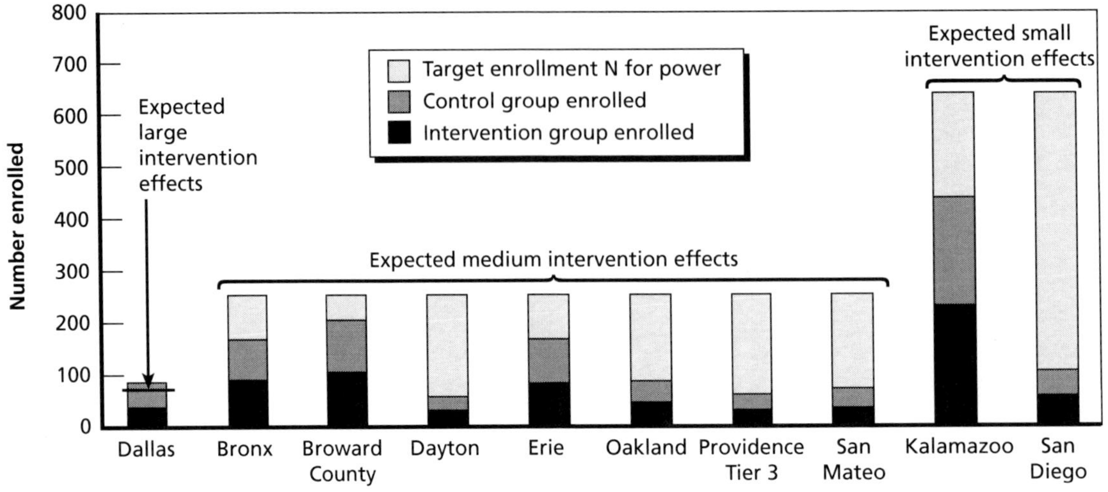

NOTE: Washington Heights/Inwood is omitted from this figure because the site did not adhere to the randomization procedures.
RAND *TR991.1-6.1*

Figure 6.2
Required Versus Actual Enrollment for Sites with Comparison Groups

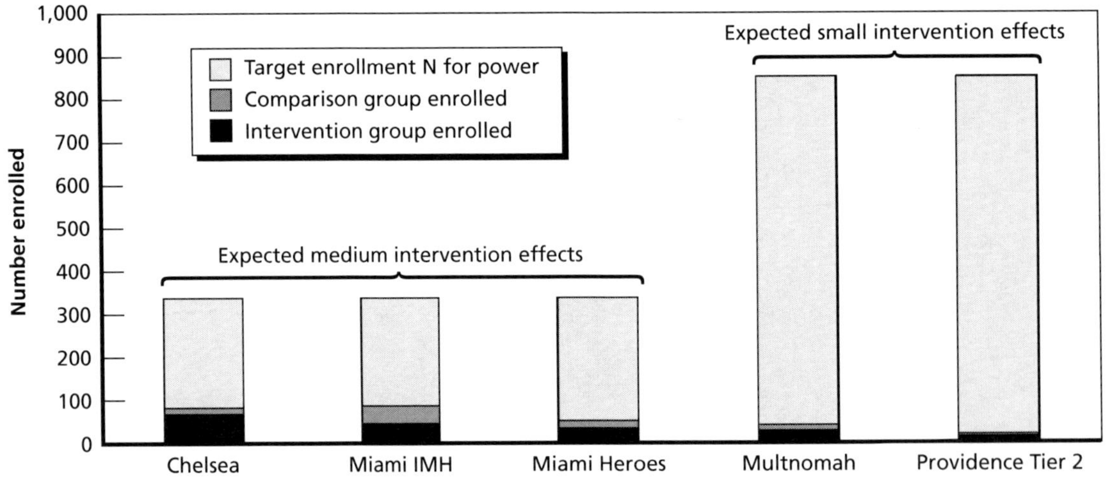

RAND *TR991.1-6.2*

Safe Start program and both Miami programs, we expected a medium intervention effect, which meant that a total of 338 families were needed to have an 80-percent chance of detecting a medium intervention effect (assuming an 80-percent retention rate). Both Chelsea and the Miami IMH program enrolled about one-quarter of the families needed, while the Miami Heroes program enrolled only 15 percent of the 338 needed. For Multnomah County and Providence Tier 2, each program enrolled approximately five percent of the total 850 families needed to have an 80-percent chance of detecting a small intervention effect (assuming an 80-percent retention rate).

Overall, the sites struggled with enrollment for multiple reasons, which are spelled out in detail in *National Evaluation of Safe Start Promising Approaches: Assessing Program Implementation* (Schultz et al., 2010). Despite efforts made to provide training and conduct outreach with referral agencies or prior experience working with the referral sources, most of the sites had a slower-than-expected pace of referrals throughout implementation. Several sites experienced difficulties with the agencies or organizations that were providing referrals into the program. For example, staff turnover at the referring agencies made it difficult to maintain the flow of referrals, since new staff were not familiar with the program or referral process. At other sites, the referral sources considered identifying and referring for violence exposure secondary to the agency's own services to the family. Similarly, at some sites, referral agency staff found it necessary to build relationships and establish trust with families before starting a discussion about violence exposure and its potential impact on children. The research context sometimes complicated enrollment for sites with randomized control designs because some referral sources were reluctant to refer families, knowing that families in the control or comparison group would not receive the program. The structure of the referral process itself also provided challenges. At some sites, the referral process was either new or cumbersome, making it difficult to develop and maintain a steady pace of referrals.

The program setting factored into enrollment as well. Some sites had smaller-than-expected pools of potential participants. For example, several of the programs operated within or took referrals directly from domestic violence shelters, which had limited capacity to serve families because of the size of the shelter or the families' lengths of stay (e.g., Dallas and Miami).

In addition to the challenges outlined above, a particular problem for sites with quasi-experimental designs was the difficulty in enrolling a comparison group. Several of the sites that employed this design had very low enrollment into their comparison groups, such that some of the comparison groups were not usable in the outcomes analyses. These included Chelsea, Miami Heroes, and Providence Tier 2. For these sites, the staff at the agencies or programs serving as the comparison group center were reportedly not invested in identifying potentially eligible families. Further, many caregivers were difficult to locate, either initially or after enrollment had occurred.

Finally, the evaluation ended early because of funding constraints when the federal appropriation for Safe Start was curtailed. The sites were fully funded for four years of program implementation, starting in October 2005 and ending in September 2009. It was expected that the sites would enroll families in the studies over a 3.5-year period (42 months). Because of the varying length of the start-up period, the implementation time lines were staggered across the sites. When the funding for the national evaluation ended prematurely after four years instead of the planned five years, this meant that study enrollment had occurred over varying time frames. As shown in Figure 6.3, the shortest study enrollment period was 25 months, in San Diego, and the longest period was 44 months, in San Mateo. Most of the sites except Kalamazoo enrolled families in the study for less than the expected 42 months because of the national evaluation funding ending prematurely. Kalamazoo had completed its proposed three years of data collection by the time it ended. The three sites with the longest enrollment periods (the Bronx, Dallas, and San Mateo) were able to extend enrollment beyond the funded period by leveraging existing resources.

As noted earlier, three of the sites had more success with enrollment than the others: Broward County, Erie, and Kalamazoo. Broward County enrolled 80 percent of the 250 families

Figure 6.3
Months of Study Enrollment by Site

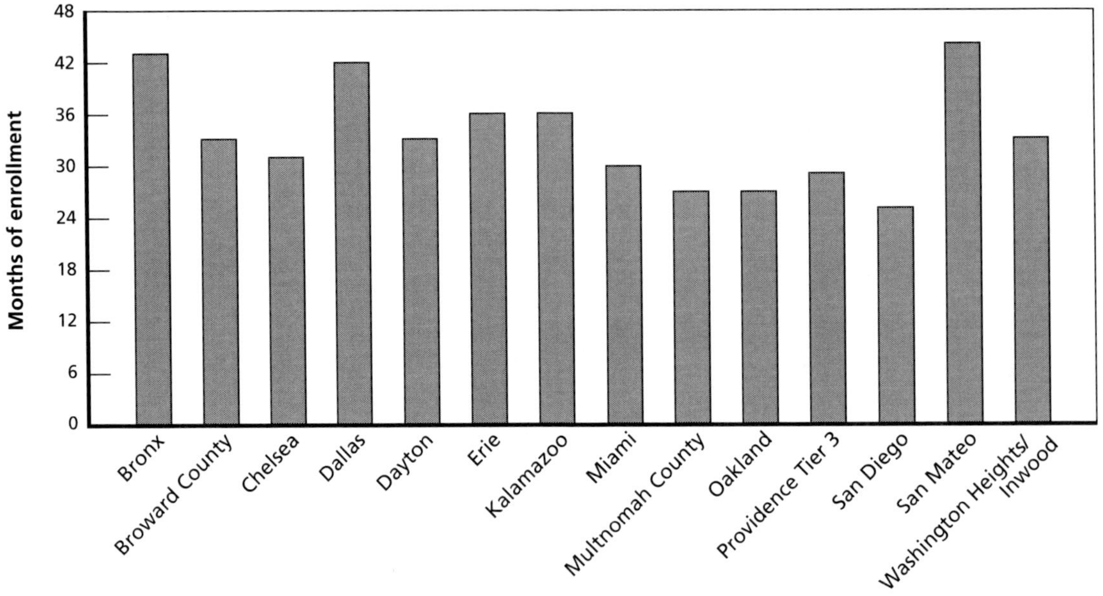

RAND *TR991.1-6.3*

needed to have an 80-percent chance of detecting a medium intervention effect (assuming an 80-percent retention rate). Broward's Safe Start program staff undertook a series of efforts to develop and maintain a steady stream of referrals, which appeared to be key to their success. These efforts included conducting ongoing trainings and informal discussions with the community workers who made referrals to increase their familiarity and comfort with the intervention, revising the program materials to make them more appealing to referring agencies and eligible families, and developing a detailed protocol for providing referrals and support to families assigned to the control group. For Erie, which ultimately enrolled 66 percent of the families necessary for power to detect the minimum observable intervention effect, the pace of recruitment and enrollment during the first year was much slower than the program expected. Initially, the referral sources were either not referring families or not referring enough families to meet the needed enrollment numbers. Partway through implementation, the Erie project team developed a multipronged approach to increasing referrals and enrollment that included increasing the target child age range, conducting outreach to some of the places that were not referring at all, providing education for the agencies that were referring, and promoting Safe Start internally within the Children's Advocacy Center. Together, these efforts dramatically increased referrals and enrollment.

Kalamazoo enrolled 68 percent of the children necessary to have the power to detect a small intervention effect, assuming an 80-percent retention rate. The mechanics of recruiting children from Head Start classrooms appeared to be a good strategy for enrolling families, and recruitment was limited only by staffing constraints on the number of classrooms that could be included. Safe Start program staff screened students within Head Start themselves, after families expressed interest in participating. This alleviated some of the burden on the Head Start staff and ensured that most families within Head Start were approached about participating in the study. Kalamazoo also created a community workgroup focused on violence, convening it for the first 18 months of the project, until the relationships among agencies and with Head Start were well established.

Summary of Retention Across Sites

The outcome evaluation was further constrained by attrition at each site, which reduced the sample size in the study even at sites that had been able to initially enroll families nearing the target for power. Figure 6.4 shows the average retention rates for the six-month assessments by site. Although, theoretically, attrition that happens completely at random will not have any impact on the external validity of inferences made, attrition can often be related to treatment factors leading to selection bias. Thus, generally it is good practice to target an 80-percent retention rate in intervention research with the hope of avoiding any possible selection bias. Only Kalamazoo, Chelsea, and San Diego reached an 80-percent retention rate at six months.

Figures 6.5 and 6.6 show the samples retained for the six-month assessment for sites with randomized control trials and comparison groups, respectively. As noted above, one site (Dallas) enrolled enough families to have an 80-percent chance of detecting the expected intervention effect. However, Dallas only retained approximately one-half of all enrolled families at the six-month assessment point, meaning that the size of the retained sample fell well below the sample size needed for the power to detect the minimum observable effect.

Low retention rates created two other issues that affect the interpretation of findings. First, low retention can create biases in the sample, such as when families in more distress are more likely to leave the study and be lost to follow-up. In such cases, the results can be misleading, and the impact of attrition on the balance across the groups should be examined. Low retention is a definite issue for sites that retained less than 50 percent of the original sample,

Figure 6.4
Six-Month Retention Rates

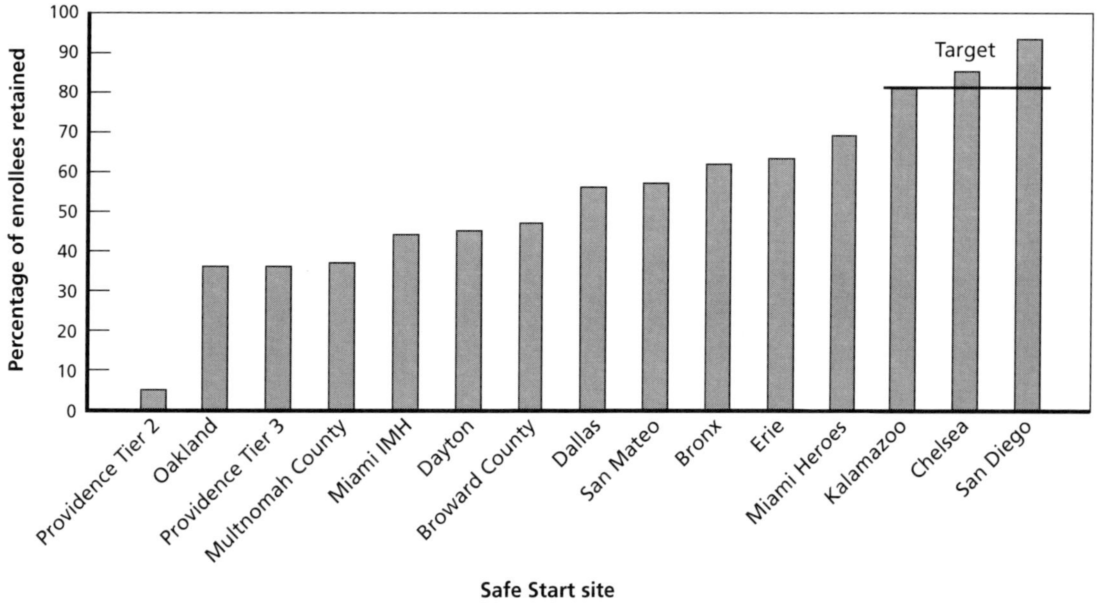

RAND *TR991.1-6.4*

Figure 6.5
Six-Month Retention for Sites with Randomized Control Trials

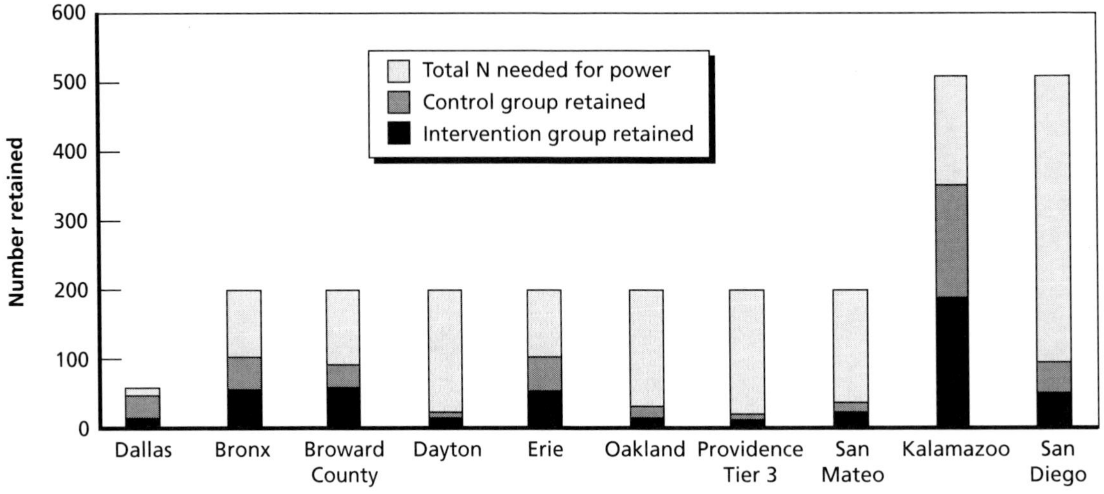

RAND *TR991.1-6.5*

Figure 6.6
Six-Month Retention for Sites with Comparison Groups

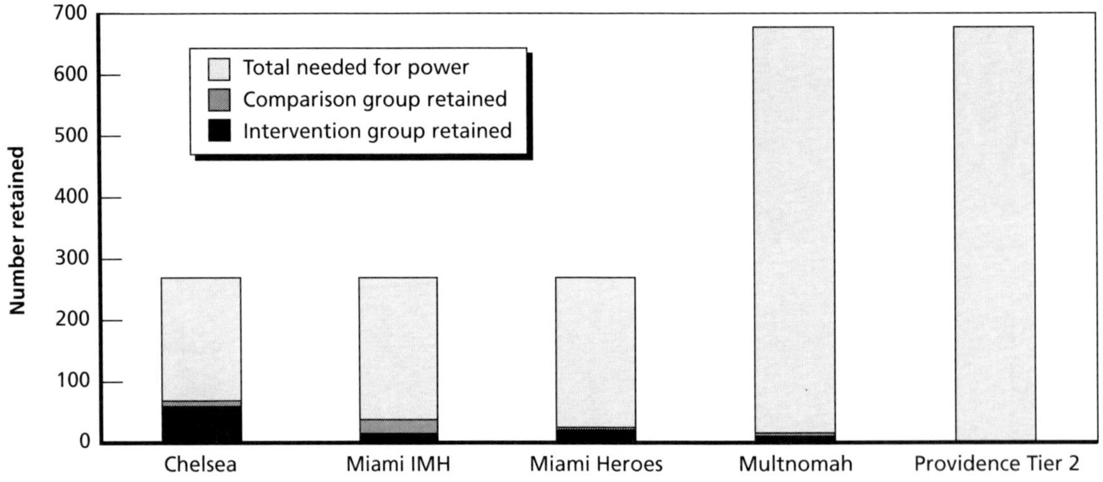

RAND *TR991-6.6*

including Broward County, Washington Heights/Inwood Kids' Club, Providence, Oakland, Multnomah County, Miami IMH, and Dayton, increasing the potential for biased results from these sites.

Secondly, differential retention between the two groups, such as when families in the intervention are retained with higher frequency than families in the control group, can also bias the results. This was the case in several sites, including Dallas, San Mateo, Miami Heroes, and Broward County. We conducted an additional analysis in Dallas and Broward County, contrasting the baseline measured characteristics of children retained at six months to children who dropped out before six months, and found no evidence of systematic differences in outcome measures or demographics at baseline between the groups of children retained versus those who dropped out in these two sites. However, in the other sites the number of participants was too small to explore this issue.

Several sites had success with retention, achieving the target 80-percent retention rate for the six-month assessment. In Chelsea, the health clinic setting meant that families were coming to the clinic for other appointments, not just for the research assessment. This provided the Safe Start program staff with multiple opportunities to complete the assessments. Kalamazoo hired retired social workers on a contractual basis to collect follow-up assessments. These staff members had a high level of comfort in working with impoverished families and went to family homes to conduct the assessments. The assessors made multiple attempts to find families and could devote all their energy to the task, as they were employed solely for the purpose of completing them. In San Diego, once families were enrolled, the site was able to maintain a very high rate of retention in the study, which is attributed to regular contacts with families to confirm contact information, multiple methods of contacting families to schedule assessments, and flexibility in scheduling follow-up assessments. We note, though, that it is likely that successful retention was influenced by other factors as well, as sites that achieved lower retention rates also employed similar strategies to those listed here.

Summary of the Power/Design Issues Across Sites

Overall, because of issues with underenrollment and attrition and the premature end of the evaluation, in most sites the retained sample was smaller than the sample needed for power to detect the minimum observable effect. That is, most of the studies were underpowered for the evaluation. We therefore explain in each site report the chances of detecting the expected intervention effect, given the sample in the study, as a way of interpreting the findings within each evaluation. We will organize the review of findings into three categories of sites, based on their final designs and sample sizes.

Five sites were marginally powered to examine the potential impact of the program (Kalamazoo for a small to medium effect; Broward County, Bronx, and Erie for a medium to large effect; and Dallas for a very large effect). For these sites, we expected that we might be able to observe intervention effects if the effects were in the range expected, but the intervention effects would have to be slightly larger than any anticipated to have more than an 80-percent chance of detecting them.

On the other hand, several sites were clearly underpowered for detecting intervention effects, including the small intervention effects expected in San Diego and medium intervention effects expected in Miami IMH, Dayton, Oakland, Providence Tier 3, and San Mateo. For these sites, we did not expect to be able to detect intervention effects, if they existed, given inadequate power.

Third, some sites completely lacked an adequate control/comparison group, including Chelsea, Multnomah County, Washington Heights/Inwood CPP and Kids' Club, Miami Heroes, and Providence Tier 2. For these sites, no inferences can be drawn about the impact of the programs. Futhermore, for Providence Tier 2, the sample size in the intervention group was also small, limiting the power to test for within-group changes as well.

Overview of Findings

The main findings from the 15 studies are found in Results Appendixes A–O, presented in alphabetical order by site name. Here, we organize the overview of findings from the study into three groupings, according to our ability to draw firm inferences from the studies about intervention effects. Of note in the evaluation is the fact that many within-group changes in the outcomes variables were observed over time in the intervention groups, showing movement in the direction of improvement in symptoms, behaviors, or violence exposure. However, there were also often improvements noted in the control groups for these sites, such that there was no overall difference in differences observed in most cases between the intervention and control/comparison conditions on improvements in symptoms, behaviors, or violence exposure.

In the first category are programs that were marginally powered to detect intervention effects in the general range we expected. For these, the data generated can give some indication of the promise of the programs, but the intervention effects would need to be somewhat larger than originally expected to have a high probability (>80 percent) of detecting them. Five sites fit into this category, including the Bronx, Broward County, Dallas, Erie, and Kalamazoo. All but one of these sites delivered interventions that lasted about six months, and thus the six-month assessment would give the most robust test of outcomes. The Bronx model lasted 12 months or more, and so we also examine 12-month outcomes for that site. In general, both the intervention and control or comparison groups showed significant improvements in outcomes between baseline and six months. In some cases, significant improvements were seen in the intervention group but not in the control group. These included caregiver report of child PTSD symptoms (Erie and Kalamazoo), aspects of parenting stress (the Bronx, Erie), aspects of social emotional competence (the Bronx, Broward County, Erie, Kalamazoo), caregivers' personal problems (Dallas), and aspects of academic achievement (Kalamazoo). At 12 months, this pattern of results persisted in the Bronx and also included child behavior problems. In other cases, significant improvements were seen only in the control or comparison groups but not in the intervention group, as in the case of several outcomes for Dallas at six months and PTSD symptoms at the Bronx at 12 months. In only two cases did the change in outcomes in the intervention group differ significantly from changes occurring within the control or comparison group at six months. In Erie, there was a significant improvement attributable to participation in the intervention in one of the 18 primary outcomes identified, but it did not remain significant once demographics were controlled. In Dallas, there was a significant difference in changes in traumatic events experienced by caregivers, such that caregivers in the control group reported more substantial decreases than in the intervention group. At 12 months, two significant differences were observed in the Bronx between groups, but they operated in opposite directions and did not remain significant once demographics were controlled. In Dallas, at the 12-month mark, intervention group caregivers reported experiencing significantly less parental distress compared with caregivers in the control group. However, the sample size did not allow for analyses controlling for multiple demographics. Still, an exploratory analysis conducted controlling only for child gender shows that the difference was no longer significant once gender was controlled. For other outcomes, improvement was observed in both the intervention and control groups, particularly in terms of reductions in violence exposure for both the child and caregiver. However, these changes result partly from the time frame used in those scales, with lifetime violence exposure being assessed at baseline, and violence only during the time since baseline being assessed at the six-month or 12-month assessments.

Examination of the intensity or dosage of the interventions delivered is also important to consider in these studies. As interventions were delivered in real-world community settings, those families assigned to receive intervention services received them in varying amounts and combinations. Thus, the intent-to-treat analysis in this study, while the most valid test of the intervention, is conservative. Specifically, the intervention groups contained some individuals who received no services or very few services, and it was the minority of families that received the full intervention as designed in many of the sites. We used several different methods to examine this issue and presented the site-specific method in the site reports when the number of participants was large enough to support it. In these analyses, we compared those in the intervention group who received differing amounts of services to matched families from the comparison group who received none. We did not observe any obvious patterns in the data to suggest that receiving more of the intervention was related to a larger intervention effect but did not have sufficient power to be certain that such a relationship does not exist.

In the second category are sites that are underpowered, and thus we cannot expect to observe the size of intervention effects that the program is likely to produce. For these studies, a lack of significant intervention effects has little meaning, and we cannot know for sure whether the intervention was effective because we did not have enough power to detect the expected effects. The sites in this category included Dayton, Miami IMH, Oakland, Providence Tier 3, San Diego, and San Mateo. In these sites, significant improvements in outcomes were observed between baseline and six or 12 months for some outcomes within the intervention group, but not in the control group. These included caregiver report of child PTSD symptoms (San Diego), child behavior problems (San Diego), aspects of social emotional competence (Oakland), and caregivers' personal problems (Miami IMH). Improvements were also observed in both the intervention and control or comparison groups on the child and caregiver violence exposure measures. As expected, we did not observe intervention effects for these programs.

Finally, in the third category are sites that did not have a viable control or comparison condition, so that inferences about the impact of the program cannot be made. These include Chelsea, Miami Heroes, Multnomah County, Providence Tier 2, and Washington Heights/Inwood. Although the Chelsea program showed significant improvements on several measures, no conclusions about the intervention effects relative to a control/comparison condition are drawn. Reductions in violence exposure were also observed in these sites but were expected, given the changes observed in the other sites under study in this project for both the intervention and control or comparison groups.

Overall, the evaluation produced a large number of inconclusive findings about the impact of interventions on child-level outcomes. This may certainly be due to the lack of adequate statistical power for most sites (accentuated by the low retention rate) or the lack of an adequate control/comparison group for several sites (i.e., Chelsea, Miami Heroes, Multnomah County, Providence Tier 2, and Washington Heights/Inwood). However, there are a number of other potential explanations as well. Where adequate sample sizes did exist to allow for statistical tests (the Bronx, Broward County, Dallas, Erie, and Kalamazoo) and no statistically significant differences were found, it is possible that the interventions as implemented in these studies were simply not effective. It could be that the program services as they were delivered did not impact the population of families under study or that the dosage of the services for intervention group families was inadequate on average to produce the expected outcomes. This possibility cannot be ruled out, but these findings should not be taken as firm evidence of that conclusion either.

The inability to detect significant differences between the groups may also have been due to the particular outcomes measured. That is, programs may have improved the lives of children and families in ways that were not measured (or were measured inadequately) in this study. In choosing measures for this study, we used several criteria (as outlined in Chapter Three) so that we could maximize the likelihood of detecting important changes in child outcomes. However, the measures were uniform across the 15 sites, rather than tailored to each site. This approach may have resulted in some measures not being finely tuned enough to programs at certain sites. Indeed, some sites, such as the Miami IMH program, augmented the national evaluation with their own measures and plan to analyze them separately.

Another possibility has to do with the therapeutic process and the timing of assessments. Several sites noted that sometimes families were not aware of the connection between violence exposure and their child's symptoms at the time of entrance into the program and only became aware of this link as they learned more in the intervention process. If true, this could mean that subsequent reports of child behavior and symptoms could be heightened as compared to baseline because the caregiver is more aware and sensitive to them, and thereby they could obscure any intervention effects. Similarly, some interventions could exacerbate symptoms before reducing them, as part of the therapeutic process. If so, it would only be the later assessments (12, 18, or 24 months) that would show the full impact of the program, and the six-month assessments could be misleading.

For some sites (i.e., Broward County, Dallas, Erie), the control group received enhanced services during their involvement in the study. These enhanced services provided assurance that families' basic needs were being met, and the community partners were generally satisfied that the study was ethical and that families would be taken care of. However, the enhancements may have also served to reduce the amount of difference between the two groups and thus made an intervention effect in the absence of these enhanced services more difficult to detect.

For some sites (Broward County, Dallas, Miami Heroes, and San Mateo), differential retention in the two groups may mean that selection bias played a role in the outcomes observed. In all four sites, there was a large difference in the percentage of families retained across the groups, which could mean bias in one or both of the groups. For example, families who were having difficulty may have been more difficult to reach and assess, thereby biasing means in those assessed. Another possibility is that intervention group families were unable to engage in the services because of extremely challenging life circumstances or a mismatch between their perceived needs and the services provided by the program.

Finally, in the case of Kalamazoo and Miami IMH, participants had low levels of symptoms reported at baseline, and this may have made it difficult to demonstrate changes in children over time, since there may not have been "room" to improve for children who were not experiencing many symptoms or problems at baseline. Here, services could potentially provide a longer-term protective benefit that could not be observed in the current studies.

Conclusions and Implications

As focus on children's exposure to violence has increased among researchers and public agencies, and its negative consequences on health, behavior, and development have become more evident, intervention programs have been developed to try to improve outcomes for these children. However, many of these programs lack evidence of efficacy or effectiveness on child-level outcomes, and the few that have been empirically evaluated have not been well tested in community settings. As such, the evaluations conducted as part of the SSPA are important, as they attempt to rigorously examine the effectiveness of such programs delivered in community settings. Eighteen different evaluations within 15 sites were launched, all utilizing experimental or quasi-experimental designs, with 13 of the 18 evaluations attempting to conduct randomized controlled trial designs and the remaining five recruiting community comparison groups. This level of rigor is rarely seen in real-world implementation projects. It is particularly noteworthy in evaluation of interventions for children, where issues related to informed consent and participation tend to be more complex. Further, the complexity increases when the focus is on violence, where the sensitivity of the data collected is particularly high.

The diversity of the SSPA programs under study is also noteworthy. Although the programs all focused on children exposed to violence, they varied considerably in terms of the type of intervention, the setting in which it was offered, and the group of children and families targeted for the intervention. Sites addressed multiple forms of violence exposure and assessed exposure to all types. All of the programs were able to successfully launch and provide some services to children and families exposed to violence, as detailed in our report on SSPA implementation (Schultz et al., 2010).

Obstacles to the successful evaluation of these programs were numerous, and some of them were at least partially surmounted. For instance, finding measures that could assess these sensitive topics and examine outcomes on a wide age range was accomplished by capitalizing on the research literature, consulting and collaborating with sites on the choice of measures, working with multiple IRBs to assure confidentiality of the data collected and the limits to confidentiality, and using advanced psychometric techniques to develop measures that would span a broader age range. Second, engaging community partners and families into evaluation studies was accomplished through use of evidence-based engagement practices (McKay and Bannon, 2004) and work on messaging about the programs and evaluation, such that many families and community partners accepted randomization when that was part of the research design. Some sites were particularly successful in recruiting families into the programs in this manner, and some were quite successful in retaining them in the follow-up study assessments.

Other obstacles were harder to overcome. For instance, the funding for these projects was relatively modest, and the funding for data collection activities was limited. This made it difficult for sites to expand their services enough to have a study size adequate for a fully powered study. Moreover, the curtailment of the funding for the SSPA initiative partway through the project also made it impossible to extend data collection to make up for slow enrollment in the beginning of projects. Second, families did not always receive the interventions as intended, sometimes leaving services early, meaning that families received fewer services than would be preferred or initially intended and possibly dampening any intervention effect that could be observed. Finally, some sites struggled with recruitment and/or retention, weakening the ability to draw firm conclusions from the data collected.

Despite the limitations, these data will be useful in planning future research endeavors. Data of this type are needed in planning research efforts in community settings, in order to estimate variability around outcomes in intervention and control groups, to plan power analyses for future studies, and to understand the degree of change that might be expected in similar efforts (Leon, Davis, and Kraemer, 2010). We hope that evaluators in the future will be able to make good use of this data, which will be archived for public use according to OJJDP policy.

The difficulties faced in conducting this outcome evaluation will also provide useful information about the types of challenges faced by families entering intervention services and the challenges in evaluating child outcomes in a variety of settings. Practitioners using interventions such as these, or in these types of settings, are advised to examine this report and the process evaluation report to understand the nature of problems they might encounter and families' willingness to accept or adhere to services.

In summary, while the outcomes evaluation overall produced no conclusive findings about the effectiveness of the interventions under study, the national SSPA process evaluation identified many successes of the individual programs in implementing their program goals (Schultz et al., 2010). These successes included development of procedures for increased identification of children exposed to violence, improving communication and coordination among service providers, and establishment of new interagency and communitywide partnerships to address service gaps for children and their families. These improvements have value in their own right and should be considered as part of the legacy of the National Safe Start Promising Approaches Initiative.

References

Abidin, R. R., *Parenting Stress Index*, 3rd ed., Lutz, Fla.: Psychological Assessment Resources, Inc., 1995.

Albertus, C., J. Birkinbine, M. A. Lyon, and J. Naibi, "A Validity Study of the Social Skills Rating System—Teacher Version with Disabled and Nondisabled Preschool Children," *Perceptual and Motor Skills*, Vol. 83, 1996, pp. 307–316.

Baum, K., *Juvenile Victimization and Offending, 1993–2003*, Bureau of Justice Statistics Special Report, NCJ 209468, Rockville, Md.: U.S. Department of Justice, Office of Justice Programs, 2005.

Bell, C. C., and E. J. Jenkins, "Community Violence and Children on Chicago's Southside," *Psychiatry Interpersonal and Biological Processes*, Vol. 56, No. 1, 1993, pp. 46–54.

Benjamini, Y., and Y. Hochberg, "Controlling the False Discovery Rate: A Practical and Powerful Approach to Multiple Testing," *Journal of the Royal Statistical Society*, Series B, Vol. 57, 1995, pp. 289–300.

Berman, S. L., W. M. Kurtines, W. K. Silverman, and L. T. Serafini, "The Impact of Exposure to Crime and Violence on Urban Youth," *American Journal of Orthopsychiatry*, Vol. 66, No. 3, 1996, pp. 329–336.

Blackwell, T. L., "Woodcock-Johnson III Test," *Rehabilitation Counseling Bulletin*, Vol. 44, No. 4, 2001, pp. 232–235.

Bowen, N. K., and G. L. Bowen, "Effects of Crime and Violence in Neighborhoods and Schools on the School Behavior and Performance of Adolescents," *Journal of Adolescent Research*, Vol. 14, No. 3, 1999, pp. 319–342.

Bradley, R. H., L. Whiteside, D. J. Mundfrom, P. H. Casey, K. J. Keller, and S. K. Pope, "Early Indicators of Resilience and Their Relation to Experiences in the Home Environments of Low Birthweight, Premature Children Living in Poverty," *Child Development*, Vol. 65, No. 2, 1994, pp. 346–360.

Breslau, N., G. C. Davis, E. L. Peterson, and L. Schultz, "Psychiatric Sequelae of Posttraumatic Stress Disorder in Women," *Archives of General Psychiatry*, Vol. 54, No. 1, 1997, pp. 81–87.

Briere, J., *Trauma Symptom Checklist for Children (TSCC) Professional Manual*, Odessa, Fla.: Psychological Assessment Resources, 1996.

Briere, J., K. Johnson, A. Bissada, L. Damon, J. Crouch, E. Gil, R. Hanson, and V. Ernst, "The Trauma Symptom Checklist for Young Children (TSCYC): Reliability and Association with Abuse Exposure in a Multi-Site Study," *Child Abuse and Neglect*, Vol. 25, 2001, pp. 1001–1014.

Briggs-Gowan, M. J., and A. S. Carter, *Brief Infant-Toddler Social and Emotional Assessment (BITSEA) Manual*, Version 2.0, New Haven, Conn.: Yale University, 2002.

Briggs-Gowan, M. J., A. S. Carter, J. R. Irwin, K. Wachtel, and D. V. Cicchetti, "The Brief Infant-Toddler Social and Emotional Assessment: Screening for Social-Emotional Problems and Delays in Competence," *Journal of Pediatric Psychology*, Vol. 29, 2004, pp. 143–155.

Caselman, T. D., and P. A. Self, "Assessment Instruments for Measuring Young Children's Social-Emotional Behavioral Development," *Children & Schools*, Vol. 30, No. 2, 2008, pp. 103–115.

Cohen, J. A., A. P. Mannarino, and E. Deblinger, *Treating Trauma and Traumatic Grief in Children and Adolescents*, New York: Guilford Press, 2006.

Cowen, E. L., P. A. Wyman, and W. C. Work, "Resilience in Highly Stressed Urban Children: Concepts and Findings," *Bulletin of the New York Academy of Medicine*, Vol. 73, No. 2, 1996, pp. 267–284.

Delaney-Black, V., C. Covington, S. J. Ondersma, B. Nordstrom-Klee, T. Templin, J. Ager, J. Janisse, and R. J. Sokol, "Violence Exposure, Trauma, and IQ and/or Reading Deficits Among Urban Children," *Archives of Pediatrics & Adolescent Medicine*, Vol. 156, No. 3, 2002, pp. 280–285.

Department of Health and Human Services, Administration on Children, Youth and Families, *Child Maltreatment 2008*, Washington, D.C.: U.S. Government Printing Office, 2010.

Elliott, D., *National Youth Survey: Wave I, 1976*, Inter-University Consortium for Political and Social Research (ICPSR), 2008.

Epstein, M. H., *Behavioral and Emotional Rating Scale: A Strength-Based Approach to Assessment*, 2nd ed., Austin, Tex.: ProEd, 2004.

Epstein, M. H., and J. Sharma, *Behavioral and Emotional Rating Scale: A Strength-Based Approach to Assessment*, Austin, Tex.: ProEd, 1998.

Fantuzzo, J. W., R. A. Fusco, W. K. Mohr, and M. A. Perry, "Domestic Violence and Children's Presence: A Population-Based Study of Law Enforcement Surveillance of Domestic Violence," *Journal of Family Violence*, Vol. 22, No. 6, 2007, pp. 331–340.

Farrell, A. D., and S. E. Bruce, "Impact of Exposure to Community Violence on Violent Behavior and Emotional Distress Among Urban Adolescents," *Journal of Clinical Child Psychology*, Vol. 26, No. 1, 1997, pp. 2–14.

Fergusson, D. M., and M. T. Lynskey, "Adolescent Resiliency in Family Adversity," *Journal of Child Psychology and Psychiatry and Allied Disciplines*, Vol. 37, No. 3, 1996, pp. 281–293.

Finkelhor, D., R. Ormrod, H. Turner, and S. L. Hamby, "The Victimization of Children and Youth: A Comprehensive, National Survey," *Child Maltreatment*, Vol. 10, No. 1, 2005, pp. 5–25.

Finkelhor, D., H. Turner, R. Ormrod, and S. L. Hamby, "Violence, Abuse, and Crime Exposure in a National Sample of Children and Youth," *Pediatrics*, Vol. 124, No. 5, 2009, pp. 1411–1423.

Fitzpatrick, K., "Fighting Among America's Youth: A Risk and Protective Factors Approach," *Journal of Health and Social Behavior*, Vol. 38, No. 2, 1997, pp. 131–148.

Flanagan, D. P., V. C. Alfonso, L. H. Primavera, L. Povall, and D. Higgins, "Convergent Validity of the BASC and SSRS: Implications for Social Skills Assessment," *Psychology in the Schools*, Vol. 33, No. 1, January 1996, pp. 13–23.

Fusco, R. A., and J. W. Fantuzzo, "Domestic Violence Crimes and Children: A Population-Based Investigation of Direct Sensory Exposure and the Nature of Involvement," *Children and Youth Services Review*, Vol. 31, No. 2, 2009, pp. 249–256.

Garbarino, J., N. Dubrow, K. Kostelny, and C. Pardo, *Children in Danger: Coping with the Consequences of Community Violence*, San Francisco: Jossey Bass Inc., 1992.

Garmezy, N., "Stress-Resistant Children: The Search for Protective Factors," in J. E. Stevenson, ed., *Recent Research in Developmental Psychopathology: Journal of Child and Psychology and Psychiatry Book Supplement #4*, Oxford: Blackwell Scientific, 1995, pp. 213–233.

Garmezy, N., A. S. Masten, and A. Tellegen, "The Study of Stress and Competence in Children: A Building Block for Developmental Psychopathology," *Child Development*, Vol. 55, No. 1, 1984, pp. 97–111.

Gilbert, R., C. S. Widom, K. Browne, D. Fergusson, E. Webb, and S. Janson, "Burden and Consequences of Child Maltreatment in High-Income Countries," *The Lancet*, Vol. 373, No. 9657, 2009, pp. 68–81.

Gopalan, G., L. Goldstein, K. Klingenstein, C. Sicher, C. Blake, and M. M. McKay, "Engaging Families into Child Mental Health Treatment: Updates and Special Considerations," *Journal of the Canadian Academy of Child and Adolescent Psychiatry*, Vol. 19, No. 3, 2010, pp. 182–196.

Gresham, F. M., and S. Elliott, *Social Skills Rating System Manual*, American Guidance Service, Inc., 1990.

Gribble, P. A., E. L. Cowen, P. A. Wyman, W. C. Work, M. Wannon, and A. Raoof, "Parent and Child Views of Parent-Child Relationship Qualities and Resilient Outcomes Among Urban Children," *Journal of Child Psychology and Psychiatry*, Vol. 34, No. 4, 1993, pp. 507–520.

Grogger, J., "Local Violence and Educational Attainment," *The Journal of Human Resources*, Vol. 32, No. 4, 1997, pp. 659–682.

Hall, L., *Social Supports, Everyday Stressors, and Maternal Mental Health*, unpublished doctoral dissertation, University of North Carolina at Chapel Hill, 1983.

Hall, L., and A. M. Farel, "Maternal Stresses and Depressive Symptoms: Correlates of Behavior Problems in Young Children," *Nursing Research*, Vol. 37, 1988, pp. 156–161.

Hall, L., C. A. Williams, and R. S. Greenberg, "Supports, Stressors, and Depressive Symptoms in Mothers of Young Children," *American Journal of Public Health*, Vol. 75, 1985, pp. 518–521.

Hamby, S. L., D. Finkelhor, R. K. Ormrod, and H. A. Turner, *The Juvenile Victimization Questionnaire (JVQ): Caregiver Version*, Durham, N.H.: Crimes Against Children Research Center, 2004a.

———, *The Juvenile Victimization Questionnaire (JVQ): Child Self-Report Version*, Durham, N.H.: Crimes Against Children Research Center, 2004b.

Hurt, H., E. Malmud, N. L. Brodsky, and J. Giannetta, "Exposure to Violence: Psychological and Academic Correlates in Child Witnesses," *Archives of Pediatrics & Adolescent Medicine*, Vol. 155, No. 12, 2001, p. 1351.

Jaycox, L. H., B. D. Stein, and L. M. Amaya-Jackson, "School-Based Treatment for Children and Adolescents," in E. B. Foa, T. M. Keane, M. J. Friedman, and J. A. Cohen, eds., *Effective Treatments for PTSD: Practice Guidelines from the International Society of Traumatic Stress Studies*, New York: Guilford Publications, 2008, pp. 327–345.

Jaycox, L. H., B. D. Stein, S. H. Kataoka, M. Wong, A. Fink, P. Escudero, and C. Zaragoza, "Violence Exposure, Posttraumatic Stress Disorder, and Depressive Symptoms Among Recent Immigrant Schoolchildren," *Journal of the American Academy of Child and Adolescent Psychiatry*, Vol. 41, No. 9, 2002, pp. 1104–1110.

Kahn, R. S., D. Brandt, and R. C. Whitaker, "Combined Effect of Mothers' and Fathers' Mental Health Symptoms on Children's Behavioral and Emotional Well-Being," *Archives of Pediatric and Adolescent Medicine*, Vol. 158, No. 8, 2004, pp. 721–729.

Kendall, P. C., D. Cantwell, and A. E. Kazdin, "Depression in Children and Adolescents: Assessment Issues and Recommendations," *Cognitive Therapy and Research*, Vol. 13, 1989, pp. 109–146.

Kliewer, W., S. J. Lepore, D. Oskin, and P. D. Johnson, "The Role of Social and Cognitive Processes in Children's Adjustment to Community Violence," *Journal of Consulting & Clinical Psychology*, Vol. 66, No. 1, 1998, pp. 199–209.

Kovacs, M., "Rating Scales to Assess Depression in School-Aged Children," *Acta Paedopsychiatry*, Vol. 46, No. 5–6, 1981, pp. 305–315.

———, *Children's Depression Inventory (CDI): Technical Manual Update*, North Tonawanda, N.Y.: Multi-Health Systems, 2003.

Kracke, K., and H. Hahn, "Nature and Extent of Childhood Exposure to Violence: What We Know, Why We Don't Know More, and Why It Matters," *Journal of Emotional Abuse*, Vol. 8, No. 1/2, 2008, pp. 29–49.

Lanktree, C. B., and J. Briere, "Outcome of Therapy for Sexually Abused Children: A Repeated Measures Study," *Child Abuse and Neglect*, Vol. 19, 1995, pp. 1145–1155.

Lansford, J. E., K. A. Dodge, G. S. Pettit, J. E. Bates, J. Crozier, and J. Kaplow, "A 12-Year Prospective Study of the Long-Term Effects of Early Child Physical Maltreatment on Psychological, Behavioral, and Academic Problems in Adolescence," *Archives of Pediatrics and Adolescent Medicine*, Vol. 156, No. 8, 2002, pp. 824–830.

Leon, A. C., L. I. Davis, and H. C. Kraemer, "The Role and Interpretation of Pilot Studies in Clinical Research," *Journal of Psychiatric Research*, Vol. 45, No. 5, 2011, pp. 626–629.

Lieberman, A. F., and P. Van Horn, *Don't Hit My Mommy: A Manual for Child-Parent Psychotherapy with Young Witnesses of Family Violence*, Washington, D.C.: Zero to Three, 2005.

LONGSCAN Study, "LONGSCAN Measures: Pre–Age 4 Through Age 18 (Updated 02/01/10)," 2010. As of July 27, 2011:
http://www.iprc.unc.edu/longscan/pages/measelect/Measure%20Table%20(up%20through%20Age%2018%20Interviews).pdf

Loury, G., "A Dynamic Theory of Racial Income Differences," in P. A. Wallace and A. M. LaMond, eds., *Women, Minorities, and Employment Discrimination*, Lexington, Mass.: Lexington Books, 1977, pp. 153–186.

Luthar, S. S., D. Cicchetti, and B. Becker, "The Construct of Resilience: A Critical Evaluation and Guidelines for Future Work," *Child Development*, Vol. 71, No. 3, 2000, pp. 543–562.

Margolin, G., and E. B. Gordis, "The Effects of Family and Community Violence on Children," *Annual Review of Psychology*, Vol. 51, 2000, pp. 445–479.

Martinez, P., and J. E. Richters, "The NIMH Community Violence Project: II, Children's Distress Symptoms Associated with Violence Exposure," *Psychiatry Interpersonal and Biological Processes*, Vol. 56, No. 1, 1993, pp. 22–35.

Masten, A. S., "Ordinary Magic: Resilience Processes in Development," *American Psychologist*, Vol. 56, No. 3, 2001, pp. 227–238.

Masten, A. S., K. Best, and N. Garmezy, "Resilience and Development: Contributions from the Study of Children Who Overcome Adversity," *Development and Psychopathology*, Vol. 2, No. 4, 1990, pp. 425–444.

Masten, A. S., and J. D. Coatsworth, "The Development of Competence in Favorable and Unfavorable Environments: Lessons from Successful Children," *American Psychologist*, Vol. 53, No. 2, 1998, pp. 205–220.

Masten, A. S., and J. L. Powell, "A Resilience Framework for Research, Policy, and Practice," in S. S. Luthar, ed., *Resilience and Vulnerability*, Cambridge, U.K.: Cambridge University Press, 2003, pp. 1–28.

McKay, M. M., and W. M. Bannon, Jr., "Engaging Families in Child Mental Health Services," *Child and Adolescent Psychiatric Clinics of North America*, Vol. 13, 2004, pp. 905–921.

McGrew, K. S., and R. W. Woodcock, *Technical Manual, Woodcock-Johnson III*, Itasca, Ill.: Riverside Publishing, 2001.

Mercy, J. A., and J. Saul, "Creating a Healthier Future Through Early Interventions for Children," *The Journal of the American Medical Association*, Vol. 301, No. 21, 2009, pp. 2262–2264.

Merrell, K. W., and M. Popinga, "The Alliance of Adaptive Behavior and Social Competence: An Examination of Relationships Between the Scales of Independent Behavior and the Social Skills Rating System," *Research in Developmental Disabilities*, Vol. 15, 1994, pp. 39–47.

Mooney, P., M. H. Epstein, G. Ryser, and C. D. Pierce, "Reliability and Validity of the Behavioral and Emotional Rating Scale—Second Edition: Parent Rating Scale," *Children & Schools*, Vol. 27, No. 3, 2005, pp. 147–148.

Morris, E., *Youth Violence: Implications for Posttraumatic Stress Disorder in Urban Youth*, Issue Report from the National Urban League Policy Institute, Washington, D.C., 2009.

Muthen, L. K., and B. O. Muthen, *Mplus User's Guide*, Los Angeles, Calif.: Muthen & Muthen, 1998–2004.

Peterson, J. L., and N. Zill, "Marital Disruption, Parent-Child Relationships, and Behavioral Problems in Children," *Journal of Marriage and the Family*, Vol. 48, 1986, pp. 295–307.

Pollio, E. S., L. E. Glover-Orr, and J. N. Wherry, "Assessing Posttraumatic Stress Disorder Using the Trauma Symptom Checklist for Young Children," *Journal of Child Sexual Abuse*, Vol. 17, No. 1, 2008, pp. 89–100.

Prinz, R. J., M. R. Sanders, C. J. Shapiro, D. J. Whitaker, and J. R. Lutzker, "Population-Based Prevention of Child Maltreatment: The U.S. Triple P System Population Trial," *Prevention Science*, Vol. 10, No. 1, 2009, pp. 1–12.

Rak, C. F., and L. E. Patterson, "Promoting Resilience in At-Risk Children," *Journal of Counseling & Development*, Vol. 74, No. 4, 1996, pp. 368–373.

Reitman, D., R. O. Currier, and T. R. Stickle, "A Critical Evaluation of the Parenting Stress Index–Short Form (PSI-SF) in a Head Start Population," *Journal of Clinical Child and Adolescent Psychology*, Vol. 31, No. 3, 2002, pp. 384–392.

Rivett, M., E. Howarth, and G. Harold, "'Watching from the Stairs': Towards an Evidence-Based Practice in Work with Child Witnesses of Domestic Violence," *Clinical Child Psychology and Psychiatry*, Vol. 11, No. 1, 2006, pp. 103–124.

Rutter, M., "Meyerian Psychobiology, Personality, Development, and the Role of Life Experiences," *American Journal of Psychiatry*, Vol. 143, No. 9, 1986, pp. 1077–1087.

———, "Resilience Reconsidered: Conceptual Considerations, Empirical Findings, and Policy Implications," in J. P. Shonkoff and S. J. Meisels, eds., *Handbook of Early Childhood Intervention*, 2nd ed., New York: Cambridge University Press, 2000, pp. 651–652.

Samejima, F., "Graded Response Model," in W. J. van der Linden and R. K. Hambleton, eds., *Handbook of Modern Item Response Theory*, New York: Springer-Verlag, 1997, pp. 85–100.

Sastry, N., and A. R. Pebley, *Non-Response in the Los Angeles Family and Neighborhood Survey*, Santa Monica, Calif.: RAND Corporation, DRU-2400/7-LAFANS, 2003. As of July 27, 2011: http://www.rand.org/pubs/drafts/DRU2400z7.html

Schechter, S., and L. J. Edleson, *Effective Intervention in Domestic Violence and Child Maltreatment Cases: Guidelines for Policy and Practice—Recommendations from the National Council of Juvenile and Family Court Judges Family Violence Department*, Reno, Nev.: National Council of Juvenile and Family Court Judges, 1999.

Schene, P. A., "Past, Present, and Future Roles of Child Protective Services," *Protecting Children from Abuse and Neglect*, Vol. 8, No. 1, 1998, pp. 23–38.

Schultz, D., L. H. Jaycox, L. J. Hickman, A. Chandra, D. Barnes-Proby, J. Acosta, A. Beckman, T. Francois, and L. Honess-Morealle, *National Evaluation of Safe Start Promising Approaches: Assessing Program Implementation*, Santa Monica, Calif.: RAND Corporation, TR-750-DOJ, 2010. As of July 17, 2011: http://www.rand.org/pubs/technical_reports/TR750.html

Schwartz, D., and A. H. Gorman, "Community Violence Exposure and Children's Academic Functioning," *Journal of Educational Psychology*, Vol. 95, No. 1, 2003, pp. 163–173.

Singer, M. I., T. M. Anglin, L. Y. Song, and L. Lunghofer, "Adolescents' Exposure to Violence and Associated Symptoms of Psychological Trauma," *Journal of the American Medical Association*, Vol. 273, No. 6, 1995, pp. 477–482.

Spencer, M. S., D. Fitch, A. Grogan-Kaylor, and B. McBeath, "The Equivalence of the Behavioral Problem Index Across U.S. Ethnic Groups," *Journal of Cross-Cultural Psychology*, Vol. 36, 2005, pp. 573–589.

Squires, J., L. Potter, and D. Bricker, "Revision of a Parent-Completed Developmental Screening Tool: Ages and Stages Questionnaires," *Journal of Pediatric Psychology*, Vol. 22, No. 3, 1997, pp. 313–328.

———, "Appendix F: Technical Report on ASQ," in *The ASQ User's Guide for the Ages & Stages Questionnaires (ASQ): A Parent-Completed, Child-Monitoring Questionnaire*, Baltimore, Md.: Paul H. Brookes Publishing Co., 1999.

Thissen, D., *Multilog User's Guide: Multiples, Categorical Item Analysis and Test Scoring Using Item Response Theory*, Chicago, Ill.: Scientific Software, 1991.

Thornberry, T. P., M. D. Krohn, A. J. Lizotte, C. A. Smith, and P. K. Porter, *Taking Stock: An Overview of Findings from the Rochester Youth Development Study*, paper presented at the American Society of Criminology meeting, 1998.

Werner, E., "Resilience in Development," *Current Directions in Psychological Science*, Vol. 4, No. 3, 1995, pp. 81–84.

Wierzbicki, M., and G. Pekarik, "A Meta-Analysis of Psychotherapy Dropout," *Professional Psychology: Research and Practice*, Vol. 24, No. 2, 1993, pp. 190–195.

Zinzow, H. M., K. J. Ruggiero, H. Resnick, R. Hanson, D. Smith, B. Saunders, and D. Kilpatrick, "Prevalence and Mental Health Correlates of Witnessed Parental and Community Violence in a National Sample of Adolescents," *Journal of Child Psychology and Psychiatry*, Vol. 50, No. 4, 2009, pp. 441–450.